PANDEMIC BUSTERS
A Prepper's Handbook

Eddie Ramirez, M.D.
Cari Haus

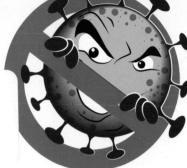

22 Simple and Easy Immune Boosters You Can Do at Home

CONTENT

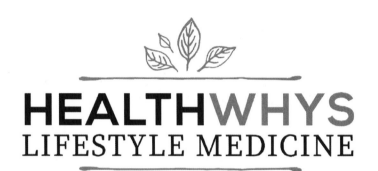

Copyright © 2021 by:

HealthWhys Lifestyle Medicine
2363 Mountain Road
Hamburg, Pennsylvania 19526

Second Printing

All rights reserved. No part of this publication may be reproduced, distributed, or transmitted in any form or by any means, including photocopying, recording, or other electronic or mechanical methods, without the prior written permission of the publisher, except in the case of brief quotations embodied in critical reviews and certain other noncommercial uses permitted by copyright law.

For permission or bulk copy requests, contact the publisher, addressed **"Attention: Permissions Coordinator,"** at this address: info@healthwhys.com or **call (610) 685-9900**, or visit our website at http://www.pandemicbusters.org/.

Cover and Interior Design: Olena Lykova

ISBN: 978-1-955866-00-2

Copyright Registration: TX 9–008–828

This book contains the opinions and ideas of its authors. It is intended to provide helpful general information on the subjects that it addresses. It is not in any way a substitute for the advice of the reader's own physician(s) or other medical professionals based on the reader's own individual conditions, symptoms, or concerns. If the reader needs personal medical, health, dietary, exercise, or other assistance or advice, the reader should consult a competent physician and/or other qualified health care professionals. The author and publisher specifically disclaim all responsibility for injury, damage, or loss that the reader may incur as a direct or indirect consequence of following any direction or suggestions given in this book or participating in any programs described in this book.

STUDY HISTORY

Or You May Be Deleted

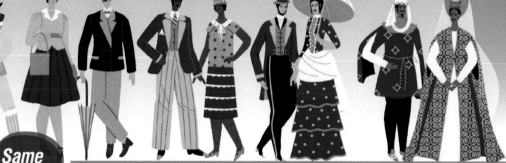

SHOULDN'T THAT BE *"Study history or you will repeat it?"*

Same thing

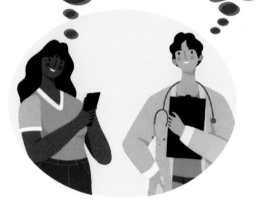

Why Flu History *(Flu-story)* Matters...

1 More pandemics are likely to come.

More than a few experts believe that COVID-19 is simply an "ugly dress rehearsal" for the big – and more deadly – pandemic yet to come. And sorry to say it, but there are plenty of reasons to believe that is true.

2 In past centuries, people have endured many pandemics.

There is much we can learn from them.

5 There were a few gleams of hope!

One college dorm that had 90 students come down with the Spanish Flu had zero fatalities — using the remedies explained in this book.

3 The Spanish Flu of 1918 was extremely deadly.

A third of the world "caught" this lethal flu, which killed more soldiers than World War I.

4 Medicine couldn't do much for this deadly flu.

Doctors and nurses stood helplessly by as patients died by the thousands. None of the normal remedies were particularly helpful.

6 Some sanitariums had an amazing track record in treating the flu!

The mortality rate for sanitariums was much lower than that of the general hospitals of the day.

7 The same remedies that worked in 1918 have been shown to work very well against COVID-19.

By studying and understanding these evidence-based, proven remedies you can build a stronger immune system which will help you:

- **Resist future viruses and pathogens**
- **Minimize the severity of any "bugs" you do catch**
- **Reduce the long-term health challenges that you might otherwise face as a result of catching a terrible virus or pathogen**

Fascinating Flu Stories & Facts

SPANISH FLU MORTALITY RATES WERE INFLUENCED BY PLACE OF TREATMENT

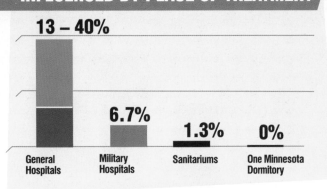

13 – 40%
General Hospitals

6.7%
Military Hospitals

1.3%
Sanitariums

0%
One Minnesota Dormitory

Some Had it Worse Than Others

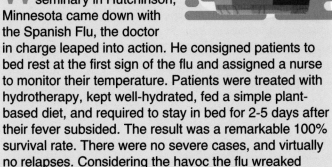

During the Spanish Flu of 1918:
- 50% of Alaskan adults perished
- 21,000 children were orphaned in New York City alone
- Young people were hit the hardest, with half of those who died being in their 20's and 30's

Recovery in a Tent

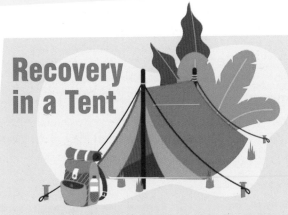

One British solder, Patrick Collins, dragged his tent up on a hill away from his regiment at the first sign of the Spanish Flu. He was one of the few from his regiment to survive – which may have been due to the fresh air, sunshine, and peaceful rest up on the hill.

100% Survival Rate

When 90 students at a seminary in Hutchinson, Minnesota came down with the Spanish Flu, the doctor in charge leaped into action. He consigned patients to bed rest at the first sign of the flu and assigned a nurse to monitor their temperature. Patients were treated with hydrotherapy, kept well-hydrated, fed a simple plant-based diet, and required to stay in bed for 2-5 days after their fever subsided. The result was a remarkable 100% survival rate. There were no severe cases, and virtually no relapses. Considering the havoc the flu wreaked elsewhere, this record was truly amazing!

Epidemics That Have Shaped History

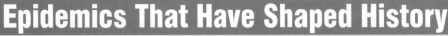

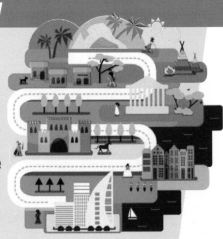

- The death of a fourth of Athenian troups due to Typhoid Fever in 430 B.C. forever shifted the balance of power between the Greek cities of Athens and Sparta.

- The Roman Empire was severely weakened twice after losing between a quarter and a third of its population to epidemics.

- The smallpox and measle epidemics that hurt the Roman empire so badly also advanced the cause of Christianity. While the pagans panicked and abandoned their sick, Christians cared for the sick of all religions. Many surviving pagans noticed this and decided to become Christians!

- Diseases brought from Europe took more native American lives than the conquerors did (90-95%).

- In 1812, Typhus infections played a major role in the destruction of Napoleon's army in Russia.

7 TREATMENTS THAT WORKED
for the Spanish Flu

The Spanish Flu pandemic of 1918 was the deadliest plague in modern times – killing an estimated 50-100 million people.

Some people were much more successful at fighting off the flu than others. Here's what the survivors did.

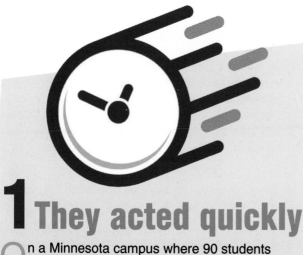

1 They acted quickly

On a Minnesota campus where 90 students caught the deadly flu, those who got sick were sent to bed pronto! Sanitariums around the country reported that the sooner they treated the patient, the higher the survival rate. People who just kept going and thought they could "beat the flu" didn't survive!

> *The best doctors give the least medicine.*
> — Benjamin Franklin

2 They went to bed... and stayed there for a while

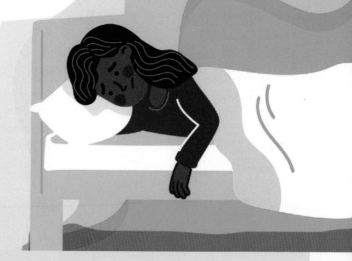

In addition to going to bed the minute symptoms began, survivors on the Minnesota campus (where 100% survived and no one even got very sick) stayed in bed 2-5 days after their fever left. The happy results? No relapses.

3 They used hydrotherapy

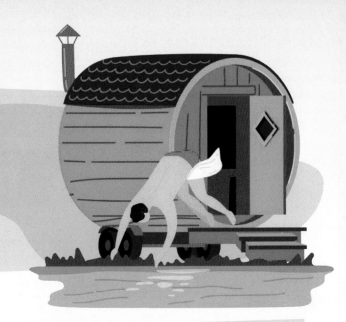

- Hot compresses were applied to the throats and chests of patients.
- You can do the same treatment today with hot showers, baths, saunas or heating pads.
- Heat kills bacteria and inactivates viruses, and moist heat is better than dry.

4 They got lots of fresh air

During World War I, wounded soldiers treated in tent hospitals had much lower mortality rates than those treated indoors. One outdoor hospital was also highly effective during the Spanish Flu. Sanitariums mimicked the outdoor treatment by having large open windows, high ceilings, and well-ventilated rooms.

5 They bathed in the sun

On nice days, tent hospitals pulled patients outside and into the sunshine. Within just one day, many of the patients who were taken outside showed remarkable improvement. Sanitariums threw open their large windows to let sunlight stream in and moved patients as close to the windows as possible.

6 They ate a simple diet

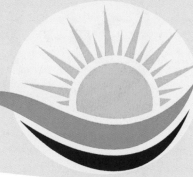

The sanitariums that had the lowest mortality rate, together with the college campus that had zero fatalities, were both serving simple, plant-based diets to the sick. Meals were light in nature, to help the immune systems of those ill to focus on fighting the flu.

7 They drank lots of water

Encouraging patients to drink plenty of water was definitely an important part of the treatment regimen at both the seminary and sanitariums.

Action Plan

→ Find ways you can get more fresh air at home and at work, and put them into action. Do the same for sunlight.

→ Consider your normal "modus operandi" when coming down with a "bug." If rest and non-drug therapies haven't been high on your list in the past, make a plan in advance to try some new things.

→ Get whatever you need – and have it on hand, for any therapies you plan to try.

GO TO BED

Find the Healing Power of Sleep

> *A good laugh and a long sleep are the best cures in the doctor's book.*
> — Irish Proverb

6 Good Things That Happen When You Get Enough Sleep

1 Your body switches into high gear and "cleans house"

Just like a parent after the kids are put to bed, your body has a whole lot of cleaning, repairing, and picking up to do while you are sleeping.

2 Your body's immune system "revs" up

Your body makes proteins that regulate cell processes (cytokines), which fortify and heal it at night.

3 The immune system's "memory" is made stronger

This helps it to "remember" how to ward off viruses and pathogens it has seen before.

4 The body's muscles and breathing activities slow down

This gives the body's defenses more energy to perform the needed maintenance.

5 More melatonin is produced

Melatonin works to reduce inflammation in the body. It also helps the body to sleep better so that it can produce even more melatonin.

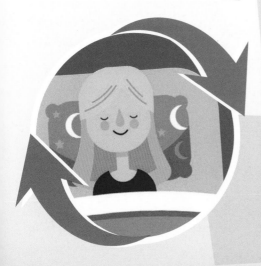

6 Sleep and your immune system help each other

- The better you sleep, the stronger your immune system.
- The stronger your immune system, the better you sleep.

Sleep is one of the most important tools to help the body ward off viruses (such as COVID-19) and other threats.

CHAPTER 2
How Pandemics Trigger
INSOMNIA

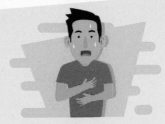

D uring a pandemic, many people experience more anxiety, fear, and/or depression than usual.

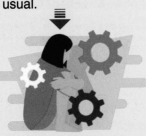

S tay-at-home orders and working at home disrupt normal routines, and with them, circadian rhythms.

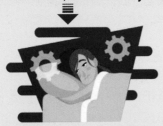

B ecause circadian rhythms regulate every cell in the body, this disruption has a negative impact on the digestion, immune response, and sleep.

When the "master clock" of the body (circadian rhythm) goes out of whack, everything else starts breaking down. The result is that insomnia – already a significant problem – becomes even worse.

Early to bed and early to rise, makes a man healthy, wealthy, and wise.
— Benjamin Franklin

Complications from Lost Sleep

- Psychological problems such as depression and anxiety
- Slower reaction time
- Lower performance
- Poor immune system function
- Obesity
- High blood pressure
- Elevated heart disease risk
- Higher risk of diabetes

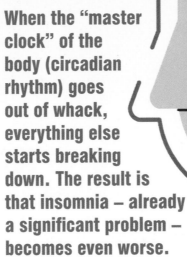

A ruffled mind makes a restless pillow.
– Old Adage

Insomnia & Depression Are Very Closely Related

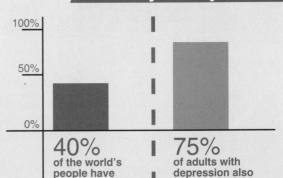

40% of the world's people have a sleep disorder

75% of adults with depression also suffer from insomnia

The Sleep-Health Connection

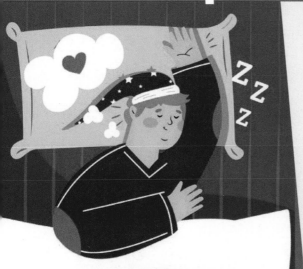

Researchers have found that:

- An extra 60-90 minutes of sleep per night makes people happier and healthier.
- People who only get 5-6 hours of nightly sleep are 4.2 times more likely to get sick than people who sleep 7+ hours.
- Those who average less than 7 hours of sleep are more likely to report being above average weight (33%), physically inactive (27%), current smokers (23%), and excessive drinkers (19%).
- People who experienced REM "dream sleep" performed 32% better at puzzle solving than those who didn't.
- Hours slept before midnight are worth much more in terms of rest than those after.
- People who sleep less than 6 hours nightly are 12% likelier to die prematurely.
- 75% of depressed individuals have chronic sleep problems, compared to 40% of adults in the general population.

WARNING:
People who get less than 7 hours of sleep each night have been shown to run a greater risk of infection.

Researchers have connected poor sleeping habits to:

- Depression
- Diabetes
- Heart disease
- Short-term illnesses

Health Benefits of Sleep

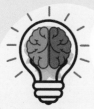

▲ IMPROVED MEMORY: Getting adequate sleep helps the brain to process new information. Sleeping soundly after you have just learned something consolidates this information into memories which are then stored in your brain.

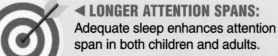

▲ REDUCED STRESS: Sleep is a powerful stress reducer. In addition to better problem-solving ability, people who are well-rested have much better coping skills.

◄ LONGER ATTENTION SPANS: Adequate sleep enhances attention span in both children and adults.

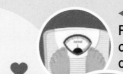

◄ HEALTHIER BODY WEIGHT: Researchers have found a close link between low sleep quality and risk of obesity.

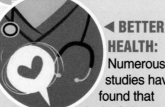

◄ BETTER HEALTH: Numerous studies have found that lack of sleep contributes to serious medical conditions. Adequate sleep does just the opposite.

◄ A HAPPIER LIFE: Research has revealed a close link between amount of sleep and overall happiness. People who are sleep deprived are much more likely to be stressed — and depressed.

► ENHANCED CREATIVITY: When you sleep, the two main phases of sleep (REM and non-REM) work together to find unrecognized links between related facts. The result of good sleep is more creativity, plus out-of-the-box solutions to vexing problems.

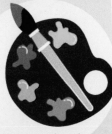

Do's & Don'ts of Healthy Sleep

Fresh Air

Walking In the Sunshine

Reading Before Bed

Nightly Routine

Meditation

Favorable Temperature

Alcohol Cigarettes

Coffee Tea

Overeating

Gadgets

TV

Stressful Events

Action Plan

→ If sleep is not a priority in your life, make and implement a plan to change that.

→ Compare your own sleep habits to the good and bad habits in the graphic above. Design and implement a plan to improve your sleep.

→ Consider and write down what health benefits you may gain by getting more and better sleep. Use this as your motivation!

RUN A FEVER
Sometimes It's Just What You Need

WERE THE GREEKS AT LEAST PARTIALLY RIGHT ABOUT FEVERS?

In ancient times, the Greeks thought fevers cured the sick by cooking the bad *"humors"* out of them. The words of Parmenides, a Greek philosopher, reflect the common thinking of his day: *"Give me a chance to create a fever and I will cure any disease."*

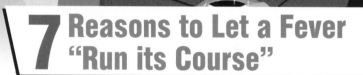

7 Reasons to Let a Fever "Run its Course"

1 Heat kills germs.

A higher body temperature performs two essential functions by:
- Stimulating the immune system
- Making survival much harder for many germs

2 Fevers speed up the body's metabolic rate.

The faster metabolic rate, in turn, revs up cell function, making the cells more efficient at fighting off "bugs."

3 Fevers ramp up antibody production.

Antibodies are immune system cells that are specifically trained to fight a particular threat the body is facing. Antibodies help the body "remember" how to ward off viruses and pathogens it has seen before.

4 Fevers trigger more white blood cell production.

White blood cells are like soldiers that fight to help the body ward off any viruses or pathogens that come its way.

5 Fevers rev up interferon production.

Interferon is a natural anticancer and antiviral substance that got its name by "interfering" when unhealthy "invaders" (such as viruses) try spreading to healthy cells.

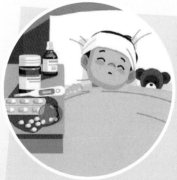

6 Letting a fever run can shorten an illness.

Studies have shown that fever-reducing drugs actually delay recovery, extending the time lost to sickness.

7 Fevers are "nature's way" to fight an infection.

Virtually all animals develop a fever naturally whenever they start to get sick. This response occurs because it gives them the very best chance to beat the illness that they are fighting. Similarly, when a virus comes knocking at your door, a fever is often just the remedy needed.

CHAPTER 3 / FEVERS AS A MEDICAL

Treatment Throughout History

- Hippocrates, the Greek physician considered by many to be the Father of Medicine, noted that malarial fever could have a calming effect on epileptics.

- Centuries later, Galen (another Greek physician) described how a case of depression was cured when the patient suffered from an attack of fever related to malaria.

- In the 19th century, the famed French psychiatrist Philippe Pinel referred to the beneficial effect of fever for psychiatric treatment in his treatise on insanity.

- During the early decades of the 20th century, artificially induced fevers were used with great success in the treatment of mental illness.

> *Fever is Nature's engine which she brings into the field to remove her enemy.*
> — Thomas Sydenham, 17th-century English physician

When you get a fever, your body is trying to turn up the heat!

- Vasoconstriction limits blood flow to the skin in an effort to conserve it for the vital organs (this is what makes the skin of a feverish person pale).
- Piloerection makes hair stand on end (another way of conserving heat for the body).
- If neither vasoconstriction nor piloerection get the job done, the body turns to shivering as a way of producing heat.

If you are fighting a "bug" and your body doesn't "gift" you with a fever, you can create your own! Intentionally raising your own temp is called

ARTIFICIAL FEVER THERAPY.

ARTIFICIAL FEVER THERAPY:

Reasons to Want it & What It Does

- Stimulates the immune system
- Improves blood circulation
- Helps eliminate toxins
- Promotes mental health
- Encourages relaxation
- Supports better and deeper sleep

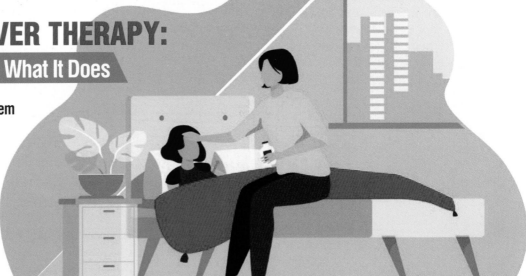

5 WAYS to Raise Body Temperature

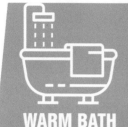

WARM BATH

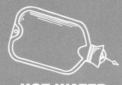

HOT WATER BOTTLE

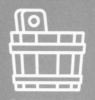

SAUNA OR STEAM BATH

HEAT WRAP, PACK OR PAD

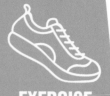

EXERCISE

THE GOAL IS TO KEEP YOUR CORE BODY TEMPERATURE AT THE BEST LEVEL FOR OPTIMAL HEALTH. IF THE TEMP IS TOO HIGH, ALWAYS TRY TO LOWER IT THROUGH NATURAL MEANS FIRST!

4 Problems Created by "Knocking Down" a Fever with Meds

1 Fever meds mask symptoms. Since people often feel better they keep going full steam when they should be resting. This has happened a lot with COVID-19.

2 Research has shown that those who take cold and fever medications are more likely to spread the virus to others.

3 It usually takes longer to recover from illness after meds have suppressed the body's immune system.

4 Lowering the fever with meds may have contributed to the cytokine storms experienced by so many COVID-19 sufferers.

The beneficial effects of a fever in fighting viruses and pathogens raise serious questions about the wisdom of taking fever-reducing over-the-counter meds for temperatures below 104° F (40° C).

SUCH DRUGS, IF CALLED UPON, SHOULD ALWAYS BE USED WITH DISCRETION.

Fevers generally do not need to be treated with medication unless your child is uncomfortable or has a history of febrile convulsions. The fever may be important in helping your child fight the infection.
— American Academy of Pediatrics

Fever Awareness Chart

	Fahrenheit	Celsius	
Low Temperature	<95°	<35°	Time to check in with your doc!
Normal Temperature	95.1-99.1°	35.1-37.3°	You're "fit as a fiddle" – or at least, your temperature is.
Light Fever	99.2-100.4°	37.4-38°	Uh oh. Time to slow down and get some rest.
Moderate Fever	100.5-103°	38.1-39.4°	Rest in earnest. Keep a careful eye on that temp. If it goes on for three or more days, seek medical help.
High Fever	103.1-105.8°	39.5-41°	Rest a lot! Try to bring the temp down through natural means. If you can't bring it down within 24 hours, seek medical help.
Very High Fever	>105.8°	>41°	Call the ambulance! You're going to the Emergency Room!

DISCLAIMER: This adult fever chart is for informational purposes only. Body temperatures will vary slightly by method of measurement. Guidelines will be different for infants, children, or individuals with underlying medical conditions. If in doubt, seek medical advice.

AN UP-AND-COMING TREATMENT FOR CANCER

HYPERTHERMIA: A cancer treatment in which body tissue is exposed to high temperatures (up to 113°F). Research has shown that high temperatures can damage and kill cancer cells, usually with minimal injury to normal tissues. This treatment is also called thermal therapy and/or thermotherapy.

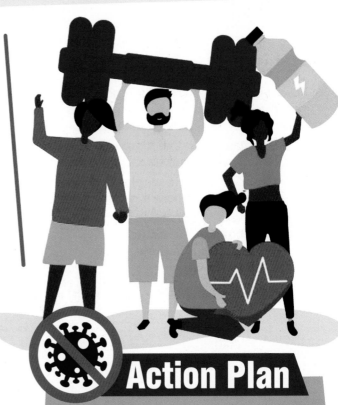

Natural Ways to Lower a Fever

- Take a tub or sponge bath using lukewarm water. Never use cold water when fighting a fever.
- Wear light PJs or clothing.
- Avoid heaping up too many blankets, even if you do have the chills.
- Drink lots of cool or room-temperature water.
- Circulate the air gently with a fan.
- Get lots of rest.
- Avoid immune-lowering foods (e.g. sugar and alcohol).

Action Plan

→ The next time you start to run a fever, think twice before taking over-the-counter medications.

→ Familiarize yourself with non-drug ways to lower a fever, and have the needed supplies on hand.

→ Consider ways that you can raise your body temperature to fight an infection, and have any needed supplies on hand.

SOAK·STEAM·DETOX
The Incredible Healing Power of Water

> *A home without a sauna is not a home.*
> – Finnish proverb

HYDROTHERAPY:
The judicious use of water to promote healing and health.

6 Things to Know about the Healing Wonders of Water

Finnish Facts About Saunas

Regular saunas are such an integral part of their culture that the Finns:

- Own more saunas per capita than anywhere else in the world (2 million, or about one per household)
- View the sauna as the "poor man's pharmacy," capable of curing many ills
- Were often (in the past) born in a sauna
- Have (in the past) used "sauna diplomacy" to negotiate with Russian diplomats.

1. Water is one of the most powerful healing agents there is. It is also the least expensive and readily available.
2. There are numerous ways in which water can aid and speed healing.
3. Many cultures have historically used some form of water (hydro) as a remedy for illness.
4. The Finns in particular are noted for their use of saunas followed by icy "plunges" as a form of treatment.
5. Because of their long experience with saunas, the Finns have accumulated an impressive body of scientific evidence documenting their health benefits.
6. Saunas are great, but you don't need one in order to do water therapy.

Some like it hot...Some like it cold...

In addition to their love for sauna heat, Finns are known for the joy they extract from icy post-sauna plunges into a lake, river, or stream. But they aren't alone...

- A Dutchman, Wim Hof, has become known as the "Ice Man" for demonstrating and proclaiming the benefits of cold water therapy.
- During the COVID-19 crisis the popularity of winter swimming, polar plunges, and "wild swims" (as winter swimming is called in Great Britain) spiraled upward worldwide.

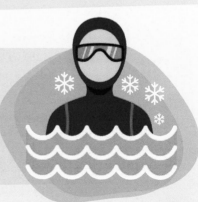

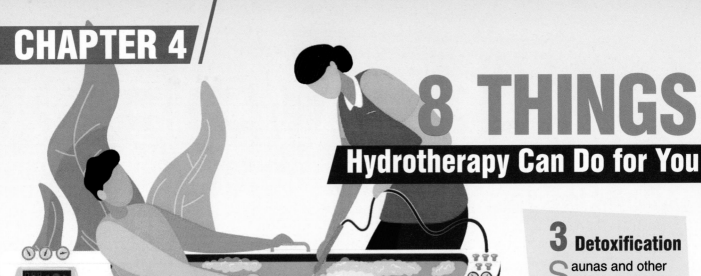

8 THINGS
Hydrotherapy Can Do for You

1 Improved Immune System Function

Hydrotherapy (whether in a sauna, bathtub, or some other form) is one of the very best ways to activate the immune system and ward off imminent threats to the body.

2 Increased Blood Circulation

At normal room temperature, about 10% of a person's blood circulates near the skin. The heat of a sauna, hot tub, or similar therapy draws about 50% of the blood to the body's surface. This action in itself causes the blood to circulate.

3 Detoxification

Saunas and other sweat-producing therapies are some of the best ways to rid the body of toxins such as dead skin cells, dirt, oil, viruses, and even heavy metals.

4 Pain Relief

When the body's deep tissues reach a temperature of about 100° F (37.8° C), nerve endings become less responsive to pain. Beta-endorphins and norepinephrine, the body's natural pain-killing agents, are also released.

5 Better Mood

Researchers have found that hot water therapy (such as saunas) boosts the body's feel-good hormones such as dopamine, serotonin, endorphins, and oxytocin.

6 Soothing of Sore Muscles

Soft, penetrating heat is very soothing to the muscles of the body. Connective tissues also become more pliant, resulting in less tension in muscles and joints.

7 Faster Metabolism

While some people argue against the benefits of hydrotherapy or a sauna for weight loss, these treatments do boost metabolism.

8 Improved Heart Function

The high heat and low humidity in a typical hydrotherapy treatment causes blood vessels to dilate, which in turn increases cardiovascular activity without an increase in blood pressure.

Polar Bear Plunges – In a Class By Themselves!

Researchers in the Netherlands have found that "polar bear plunges" (as shocking forays into icy water are sometimes called) result in:

- A rush of adrenaline which triggers production of the anti-inflammatory cytokine IL-10, which in turn inhibits inflammatory response
- Major changes in oxygen and CO2 levels which can be particularly beneficial for improving immune system function

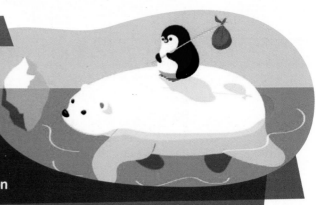

5 Easy Ways to Do Hydrotherapy at Home

No Sauna? No Problem! A sauna is just one of 5 simple ways to benefit from the healing powers of hot and/or cold water:

IMPORTANT NOTE: If your health won't allow, or you're not into the cold side of these treatments, at least do the hot. The natural chill when you finish hot treatments will result in some (though less dramatic) benefit.

METHOD №1: Take a Contrast Shower

- Try turning the hot water up as far as you can stand it without scalding.
- Stay in the hot water for about 2-3 minutes, or until you are nice and steamy.
- Turn the knob to cold for about 30 seconds.
- Repeat this 3-5 times. (You may need to build up to it!)

METHOD №2: Hop into a Hot Tub (or Warm Bath)

Hot tubs and hot baths are an excellent way to raise body temperature.

METHOD №3: Try a Thermophore®

Researchers have found that moist heat penetrates the body 27 times better than dry. One of the easiest, least expensive ways to transfer moist heat is through a hot fomentation device called a Thermophore®. These devices, which have heat controls and look like a heating pad, are inexpensive and less labor-intensive than the hot and cold compresses used in days gone by.

METHOD №4:

15-25 minutes in the sauna, followed by 30-60 seconds in cold water, is the protocol with the most health benefit. In addition to being very invigorating, the shock of the short cold treatment after the hot gives a big boost to the fighting power of the immune system.

METHOD №5: Try Fomentations

Hot and cold compresses, also known as fomentations, are another easy way to implement hydrotherapy in your home. In times past, towels used for compresses were dipped in water, wrung out, then heated on a rack over a boiling kettle of water. The arrival of microwaves made this process much easier. To make a hot compress using a microwave:

- Wet a medium-sized towel, then wring it out just a bit so it isn't overly soggy.
- Put the towel in a plastic bag and tie a knot to seal the bag.
- Place the plastic bag, with the towel inside, in the microwave and heat it for a minute or two – whatever it takes to get it quite hot.
- Use oven mitts to remove the hot towel from the bag.
- Wrap the hot, wet towel in a dry towel and apply directly to the skin on the part of the body you need to treat.

Generally, a fomentation treatment would include 3-5 minutes of hot treatment followed by 30-60 seconds of cold. This rotation would be repeated at least 3 times.

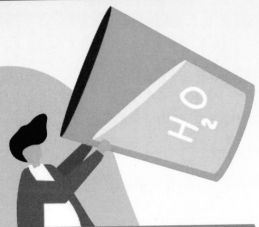

WARNING: Do not try hot-and-cold treatments if you have heart problems or arrhythmia. Although people who are physically fit can handle contrast treatments very well, the shock caused by the cold can be too much for some people.

Watch Out for These

Other considerations for anyone using hydrotherapy:

- Heat tolerance, cold tolerance, age, and vitality of the patient (special care should be taken with children, the elderly, and those who are thin)
- The room used for treatments should be warm and non-drafty
- The patient's feet should be kept warm
- After the treatment, patients should wear warm dry clothing and rest for at least 30 minutes

HOW MUCH WATER SHOULD YOU DRINK?

Answer: Enough to keep your urine clear. Another often-used rule of thumb is to drink a half ounce of water daily for every pound of body weight.

Drinking Water or "Internal Hydrotherapy" is Also Key to Good Health

HERE ARE 5 REASONS WHY:

1. **If you are dehydrated, your lymphatic system slows down.** This is very bad news, since the lymphatic system helps fight off illness-causing invaders. It also maintains body fluid levels, absorbs fats, and removes cellular waste.

2. **Drinking warm water dissolves phlegm and helps move it out of the respiratory tract.** As a result, drinking warm water can actually provide relief from a cough, sore throat, or stuffy nose.

3. **Drinking hot water helps raise the body temperature.** This, in turn, helps the body to release toxins and cleanse the blood.

4. **Drinking hot water can enhance blood circulation by breaking down fat deposits in the blood.** Cold water internally, on the other hand, can harden the oil present in food being digested. The result is fat deposited on the intestinal walls.

5. **Drinking hot water can also help to make bowel movements regular, healthy and free of pain.** A glass or two of warm water immediately upon rising in the morning can do wonders to move things along.

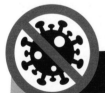

Action Plan

→ Look around your home and take note of what you have that could be used for hydrotherapy.

→ Make a plan for how you would use hydrotherapy.

→ Do a "trial run" of the hydrotherapy treatment of your choice. To boost the immune system and improve overall health, consider engaging in this hydrotherapy regularly, whether you are sick or not.

→ Consider how much water you are (or aren't) drinking. If you aren't drinking enough, think of and implement some "micro habits" that will help you to drink more water as part of your daily routine.

BREATHE TO HEAL
The Secret of Forest Bathing

In the woods, we return to reason and faith.
— Ralph Waldo Emerson

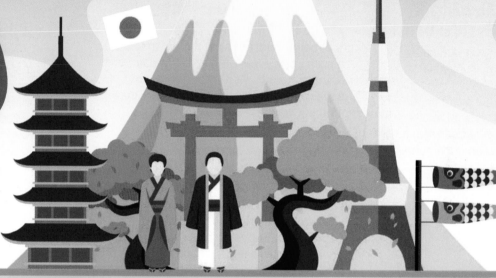

FOREST BATHING =
Spending Time Outdoors Under the Canopy of Trees

The Japanese Rediscover an Age-old Health-building Habit

- In 1982, Japan launched a national program to encourage forest bathing.

- In 2004, scientific studies of the link between forests and human health began in Iiyama, Japan, a place particularly known for its lush, green forests.

- Today, forest bathing is a popular stress management activity in that country, as more than 2.5 million people walk the trails each year as a way to relax and enhance health.

The Double Secret of the Trees

The health secrets of trees seem to lie in two things:

1. The higher concentration of oxygen that exists in a forest, as compared to an urban setting
2. The presence of plant chemicals called phytoncides — natural oils that are part of a plant's defense system against bacteria, insects, and fungi

Japanese researchers have found that exposure to phytoncides can have measurable health benefits for humans. Evergreens such as pine, cedar, spruce, eucalyptus, and conifers are the largest producers of phytoncides. That is why walking in an evergreen forest seems to have the greatest health benefits.

CHAPTER 5
7 REASONS
Why Forest Bathing is So Good for You:

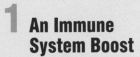

1 An Immune System Boost

In one Japanese study, subjects experienced stronger immune systems for a full week after a single forest visit. It has been documented that forests release anti-viral properties that stimulate the immune system.

2 Improved Sleep Patterns

One study found that people slept better and longer at night if they had a walk in the forest earlier in the day. Afternoon walks were reported to be especially beneficial (even more so than morning walks).

3 Stress Reduction

Evidence-based research shows that the simple act of being in the forest helps people to relax and refuel. Scientists have also found that forest therapy reduces cortisol, a stress hormone.

5 Improved Metabolic Health

Scientists have reported that forest therapy has a positive impact on adiponectin, a protein that helps regulate blood sugar levels.

6 Reduced Anxiety, Depression & Anger

The phytoncides that are present in forests, and particularly among evergreens, have been shown to help lower levels of anxiety, depression, and anger.

4 Improved Cardiovascular Health

Scientists have found that forest therapy lowers heart rates and blood pressure.

7 An Overall Boost to Health & Well-being

Researchers have found that people are "hard-wired" to respond to the natural world — so much so that the simple act of being out in nature has a profoundly positive effect on health. While other studies have shown that walking anywhere outdoors reduces depression, anxiety, and anger, Japanese scientists believe that a forest is the most beneficial place to improve vigor and energy by walking.

Fresh Air – the Elixir of Health

The abundance of pure, fresh air is a major factor behind the healing that many find in the forest. The belief in outdoor air as a remedy for many ills is actually nothing new:

- In the years before antibiotics became readily available, open air therapy was the standard treatment for many infectious diseases, including tuberculosis. Patient beds were set next to open windows in cross-ventilated hospital wards, or even placed outside.

- During World War I, casualties who were treated in open air hospitals had better survival rates, fewer infections, and speedier recoveries than those who were not.

- In Camp Brooks open-air hospital, which operated in Boston during the 1918 Spanish Flu epidemic, a much lower percentage of doctors and nurses contracted the flu than in other hospitals around the world. This much-lower infection rate was attributed to the open-air conditions at the hospital.

- In more recent times, researchers have documented that children who grow up near "green spaces" (and the fresh air they produce) have a 15-55% lower risk of developing a psychiatric illness later in life. Alcoholism, anxiety, and depression were also all associated with growing up away from "green spaces" (e.g. fields and forests).

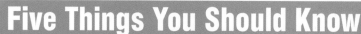

Breathe to Heal
Negative Ions:
Five Things You Should Know

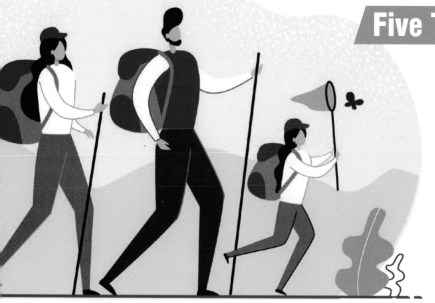

Negative Ions Are:

- Molecules floating in the air or atmosphere that have been charged with electricity
- Abundant in nature, especially around waterfalls, the ocean, mountains and forests
- Beneficial to health (as opposed to positive ions, which are not)
- One of the reasons why forests are so healing
- Present both within the air we breathe and within our bodies

Health Benefits of Negative Ions

The impact of negative ions on overall well-being and health has been scientifically proven. Researchers have found negative ions to:

- Balance the autonomic nervous system
- Enhance immune function
- Improve digestion
- Neutralize free radicals
- Promote deep sleep
- Purify the blood
- Revitalize cell metabolism

THE CURE FOR NDD (NATURE DEFICIT DISORDER)

Worldwide, the average person is said to spend 90% of their time indoors. This has a created a new, frequently diagnosed malady known (tongue-in-cheek) as NDD (Nature Deficit Disorder). Fortunately, this "trouble" can be easily cured by a simple walk through the woods!

No Forest? No Problem...

Although forests – particularly pine forests – pack an especially powerful health punch due to the essential oils, bacteria, and negative ions they produce, they are not the only place to breathe in negative ions. Here are some other negative ion-rich places to visit:

- Mountains
- Waterfalls, fountains, and springs
- Your bathroom shower
- Traditional saunas (with water poured over steaming rocks – as opposed to electric)
- Outside after a rainstorm
- Beaches with pounding surf
- Windy, moving air
- The earth (e.g. wriggling your feet in some dirt!)

NOTE: Negative ions are found mostly outside, since indoor air loses its negative polarity. Air conditioners transform negative ions into positive, which is why outside air makes such a difference in terms of clear thinking and overall health.

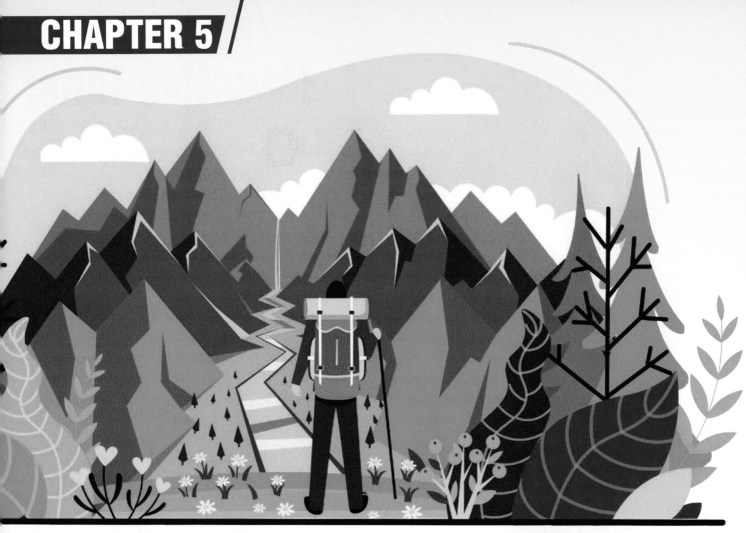

How to Forest Bathe

1. **FIND A SPOT.** You don't need to journey deep into a forest to reap the benefits of fresh outdoor air. Just look for any green area. It could be an urban park, a nature preserve, or a trail through suburban woods. Just find your happy place! The best spot for you could be a forest glade, or it could be a sunnier space.

2. **ENGAGE ALL YOUR SENSES.** Let nature enter through your ears, eyes, nose, mouth, hands, and feet. Actively listen, smell, touch, and look. Drink in the flavor of the forest, and breathe in its sense of joy and calm.

3. **DON'T HURRY.** Slow walking is recommended for beginners. It's also good to spend as much time as possible. You'll notice positive effects after twenty minutes, but a longer visit, ideally four hours, is better.

4. **TRY DIFFERENT ACTIVITIES.** You might read a book in the woods, study plants, write a poem, or find positive lessons in nature. You can venture out alone, or with a companion. In Japan, forest walking therapists are even available.

5. **APPRECIATE THE SILENCE.** One of the downsides of urban living is the constant noise. If possible, try to find a wooded area that's free from human-produced sound. Silence in itself can bring restoration. Depending on the forest, there may be many healing sounds. The rustling leaves, rippling streams, bird songs, and many other sensory blessings all help us to connect with nature, which in turn brings relaxation and peace.

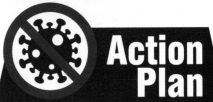 **Action Plan**

→ Think about the percentage of time you spend indoors and out. Are you struggling with "Nature Deficit Disorder"? If so, consider ways that might be changed.

→ Make a list of ways that you could be exposed to more negative ions, and decide how to get started.

→ Open your windows for 10-20 minutes daily to let the fresh air in (unless you live in a very smoggy place).

→ Make a resolution to get outside for some light exercise and fresh air at least several times daily.

GUARD YOUR NOSE:
And Entire Respiratory Tract

It All Starts With the Nose

- The nose is a major infection and transmission point for colds, the flu, and viruses such as COVID-19.

- One of the factors that made COVID-19 so deceptive and deadly was that infected people could have a virtual virus factory operating in their noses yet feel perfectly well.

- Multiple vaccine developers have recognized the importance of the nasal passage in fighting the coronavirus by focusing on nasal vaccines.

- Guarding our noses, lungs, and entire respiratory tracts is one of the most important steps we can take in the fight against viral invaders.

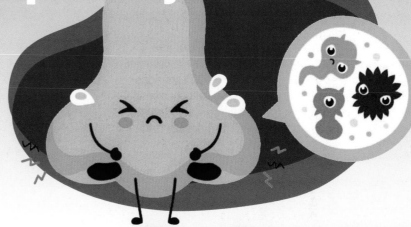

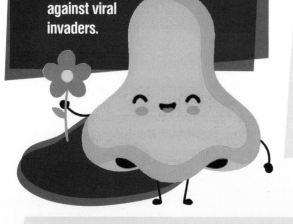

NOSE NOTES 101:
What You Should Know

- Because of its role as an air filter (removing harmful dirt and germs from air before it goes into the lungs), the nose is one of the dirtiest organs of the body.
- Mucus, which is the body's equivalent to fly paper, lines the nose in an effort to trap dirt and germs before they get to the lungs. Mucus is literally loaded with protective proteins that kill bacteria, viruses, and pathogens.
- When you blow your nose (or otherwise remove mucus from the body), you are removing the waste that mucus has "wrapped up" in an effort to protect you from infection.
- Anti-expectorants, which stop or slow the flow of mucus when you have a cold or the flu, actually work against the body's efforts to remove the infection.
- While nasal discharge may be "gross," it is an important function of your body to help you get rid of harmful viruses aand other invaders.

Your "Sniffer" is Also a "Taster"

- Those tiny smell receptors in your nose do much more than tell if refrigerated treasures are past their prime.
- The proteins used to detect certain scents (and tastes) are actually an important part of our immune system.
- Human taste buds are particularly adept at detecting the bitter, and for good reason, since most foodborne toxins are bitter to the taste.
- Researcher Dr. Noam Cohen, who went "spelunking" through the human body to see how the nose compared to the mouth and lungs, found that the same bitter-detecting taste receptors are in all three places.
- Scientists believe that the nose and lung taste receptors, which clearly aren't used for tasting, help the body to detect and fight against pathogens.

CHAPTER 6

How We Breathe

- When we inhale and exhale, the respiratory system brings oxygen into our bodies and sends carbon dioxide out.
- The exchange of oxygen and carbon dioxide that takes place when we breathe is called "respiration."

Nose Versus Mouth Breathing

- When air comes in through the nose, it is filtered, warmed, and humidified.
- Mouth breathing is not as beneficial as nose breathing since it bypasses these processes.
- Breathing through the mouth can also leave it dry, increasing the risk of bad breath and inflammation of the gums.

DIAGRAM OF THE RESPIRATORY SYSTEM

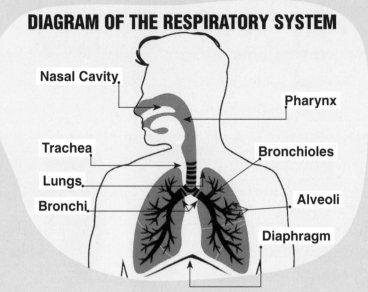

Nasal Cavity

Pharynx

Trachea

Bronchioles

Lungs

Bronchi

Alveoli

Diaphragm

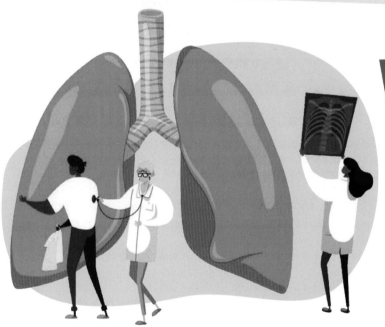

Fast Facts About the Lungs

- The surface area of your lungs is large enough to cover a tennis court
- If all of your lung airways were laid out in a line, they would cover about 1,500 miles
- Humans normally breathe at a rate of about 15 times per minute
- The average person takes somewhere near 22,000 breaths per day and inhales more than 2,000 gallons of air

What Your Lungs Do for You

When we think of the lungs, we usually think of breathing or respiration. However, the lungs perform other important bodily functions as well:

BLOOD RESERVOIR: The lungs can vary how much blood they contain at any moment, a function that is particularly useful during exercise. The lungs also work closely with the heart, helping it to function more efficiently.

FILTRATION: The lungs work to filter out small blood clots as well as small air bubbles.

PH BALANCE: The lungs protect against excess carbon dioxide in the body (which would make the body acidic) by increasing the breathing rate whenever an increase in

acidity is detected. By increasing the rate of ventilation, the lungs work to expel more of the unwanted gas.

PROTECTION: The lungs help protect against infection by secreting immunoglobulin A (an immune system antibody). The mucus in lung airways also helps to trap dust and bacteria, moving them upward to a position where they can be either coughed out or swallowed. In addition, the lungs can act as a shock absorber for the heart when physical collisions (such as an accident) occur.

SPEECH: The lungs provide airflow for speech.

4 Strategies to Keep Your Lungs Healthy

Guard Your Nose

PLEASE DON'T SMOKE

I Might Croak

STRATEGY №1:

Don't Smoke or Breathe Secondhand Smoke

- Cigarette smoke causes lung disease by damaging the airways of the lungs. Secondhand smoke will do the same.
- Smoking causes about 90% of all lung cancer deaths.
- Smoking paralyzes the cleansing mechanism of the lung (cilia).
- Because smoking impairs lung function, smokers are more vulnerable to respiratory illnesses such as pneumonia and COVID-19.

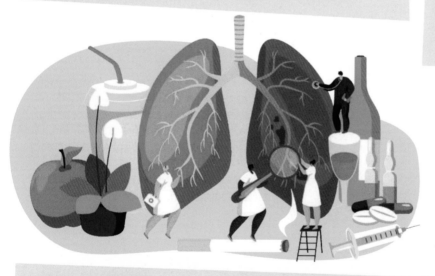

STRATEGY №2:

Avoid Breathing Lung Irritants

Environmental pollutants irritate the airways and trigger inflammation, which in turn can cause asthma attacks, chest pain, coughing, shortness of breath, or wheezing. Examples of lung irritants include:

- Artificial Fragrances
- Asbestos (a toxic chemical found in many old buildings)
- Chemical fumes, dust and mold
- Radon (a radioactive gas found in the soil)

STRATEGY №3:

Get Regular Exercise

Regular exercise can help:
- Strengthen respiratory muscles
- The body get oxygen into the bloodstream more efficiently

When you work out, your lungs exercise with you!

STRATEGY №4: Eat to Improve Lung Health

Just like other organs of the body, your lungs need healthy fuel. Nutrient-rich foods boost the immune system, which in turn wards off infection. Following is a list of seven dietary choices to avoid:

1. **ACIDIC FOODS AND DRINKS:** These can cause heartburn, which (if it occurs more than two times per week) can trigger acid reflux disease. People with lung disease often find that avoiding or limiting acidic foods (such as citrus, coffee, fruit juice, spicy foods, and tomato sauce) reduces acid reflux, and with it, lung disease symptoms.

2. **CARBONATED BEVERAGES:** Carbonated drinks cause increased gas and bloating which can put pressure on the lungs. They also contribute to dehydration.

3. **COLD CUTS:** Researchers have found a link between the nitrates in processed meats and poor lung function. These unhealthy nitrates, which cause inflammation and stress to the lungs, are found in bacon, deli meat, ham, sausage, and other processed meats.

4. **DAIRY PRODUCTS:** The casomorphins in milk increase mucus in the intestines, which can be a real problem for people struggling with lung function.

5. **EXCESSIVE SALT INTAKE:** Water retention caused by a salt-heavy diet can increase pressure on the lungs, making it harder to breathe.

6. **FRIED FOODS:** The bloating caused by grease-laden fare tends to press on the diaphragm, making breathing uncomfortable. Weight gain caused by fried food also increases pressure on the lungs, which again makes breathing more difficult.

CHAPTER 6

A Lung Disease to Watch Out For

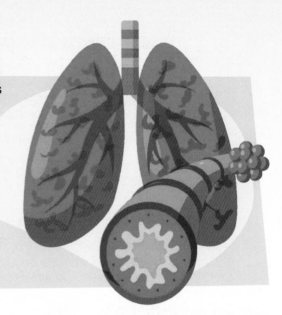

- Although lung cancer, emphysema, and COPD have been in the news for years, a serious lung disease that hasn't received as much press has gained more attention as a result of the COVID-19 pandemic.
- About 50,000 new cases of this disease, Idiopathic Pulmonary Fibrosis (IPF), are diagnosed in the U.S. each year.
- The "fibrosis" in IPF represents scar tissue in the lungs, which progresses to the point where it greatly inhibits breathing and oxygen uptake.
- Many survivors of severe COVID-19 have emerged with long-term lung damage similar to IPF.
- A deadly disease, IPF has no known cure and a median survival rate of only 2.5-3.5 years.

WHY DOES THIS MATTER?

- We should all be protecting against anything with the ability to create scar tissue in the lungs, including COVID-19, GERD, and inhaling dangerous fumes.

- The best strategy is to be proactive about our respiratory tract health by understanding how it works and continually working to enhance its function.

The GERD - IPF Connection

- In recent years, scientists have recognized a strong connection between IPF and Gastroesophageal Reflux Disease (GERD).
- An estimated 90% of people with IPF have GERD, which in turn is considered to be a risk factor for IPF.
- In a "which comes first" debate, some scientists think GERD causes IPF, while others contend that IPF triggers GERD.
- This may be because micro-aspiration of food particles into the lungs (which happens when people have GERD) can, over time, cause scar tissue in the lungs and ultimately pulmonary fibrosis.
- Researchers have found that IPF patients who managed their GERD lived about 2 times longer than those who didn't.

Let Your Nose Do Its Job

- In the 1820's, a young lawyer named George Catlin was so impressed by the healthy appearance of some Native Americans that he switched careers and spent the rest of his life documenting the habits of Native Americans.
- Catlin, who was particularly struck by the longevity and extremely low mortality rates of the tribespeople, attributed their amazing health to the tribal custom of encouraging nose breathing from infancy (among other habits).
- This early researcher believed that nose breathing led to the wider nasal passages and spectacular respiratory prowess which allowed Native Americans to lope along for miles without seeming to run out of breath.
- Catlin documented his observations in his 19th-century book "Shut Your Mouth and Save Your Life."
- Today, many are recognizing the validity of Catlin's core idea: that one of the best ways to guard our lungs and respiratory tract is to let our nose do its job — by breathing through it instead of our mouths (even during sleep).

Action Plan

→ If you have "lived with" a chronic sinus infection, try considering that in a new light. Do you really want a virtual virus factory living inside your nose?

→ Taking the suggestions made in this chapter, make and implement a plan to improve the health of your nose and entire respiratory tract.

→ If you have frequent acid reflux, or are a habitual mouth breather, give some thought as to how you can improve your habits in those areas.

HEAL YOUR GUT
Microbes Are Your Friend

YOUR GUT = YOUR DIGESTIVE SYSTEM

Hint: If it's not healthy, you won't be either.

7 Important Facts You Should Know About Your Gut

1 About 40 trillion organisms live in your gut!

The human body has so many bacteria that we've been called "walking blobs of bacteria." Yeast, fungi, and parasites are also all in the microbial mix. Other troublemakers that love snuggling into your gut include:

- Bacteriophages (teeny tiny virus monsters that infect and consume good bacteria)
- Archaea (acid-loving microorganisms that produce methane gas, which is then released when you "break wind")

2 The mini-ecosystem living in your gut, or "microbiome" as it is called, is very similar to that of your mother's.

Babies born naturally are first inoculated with their mother's microbiome when they pass through the birth canal. The connection doesn't end there. Researchers have discovered that, your personal gut microbiome, which is very unique to you, will be most similar to that of your mother (followed by your siblings). So all that talk about pre and post-natal influences isn't bogus after all. As for family resemblances, they reach right down into our guts!

3 The microbiome in your gut has "evolved" since you were a child, and can still change.

Before birth, babies don't have much of a gut microbiome at all. After the birth canal inoculation, a child's microbiome is largely influenced by diet and hygiene over the first seven years of life. The exposure to other bacteria (e.g. playing in the dirt or with household pets) also strengthens the gut microbiome. The foundation for a child's microbiome is deeply impacted by where he or she lives and other lifestyle factors. While gut flora and fauna can be improved later in life, it will always keep a "microbial fingerprint" from those early first years — which makes them very important.

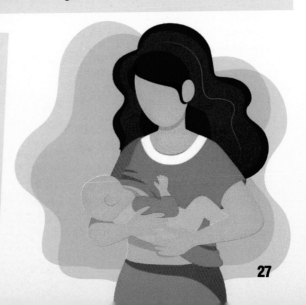

4 Your gut microbiome has a huge impact on your brain.

Your gut microbiome affects your mood, happiness, motivation, and even mental performance. That's because about 90% of the serotonin, or "happiness neurotransmitter" in your body, is produced by the microbes in your gut. Then there's the "vagus nerve," through which the bacteria in your gut is in constant communication with the brain. While this might sound a bit scary, the good news is that you can control a lot of what goes on in your gut, and the impact it has on your thinking processes, by what you eat! That's why the gut has been called the "second brain."

5 There's a "bacterial battle" raging within your body.

- The "good guys" and "bad guys" are waging a war in your gut.
- When the "good guys" have the "bad guys" in check, the body's ecosystem is in balance and all is well. But when the "bad guys" overrun the "good guys," disease is knocking at the door.
- The "bad guys" may be bacteria, viruses, pathogens, parasites, or other infectious agents.
- The "good guys" are white blood cells and good bacteria, which fend off viruses much the same way as a security detail would fight off a band of thieves.
- Your body's natural defense, which was designed to stave off disease-promoting invaders, is called the immune system.
- Infections are simply a battle between invading harmful organisms and the "good guy defenders" within your body.

6 Your gut's composition is a good predictor of whether you're chubby or lean.

Researchers have found that, when they look at a person's gut microbiome, they can tell with 90% accuracy whether that person is chubby or lean. This leads to fascinating implications for those who are overweight, in terms of the impact of making diet and lifestyle changes that positively affect the chemistry of the gut.

7 Your gut function determines how well your body is nourished.

The health of your gut microbiome affects how well your body extracts energy and nutrients from the food you eat. A healthy gut has also been closely tied to a healthy metabolism.

Watch Out for Your "Weak Spots"

- Near the end of the day, many people feel tired and exhausted.
- This state of exhaustion weakens the immune system.
- Sensing this weakness, fungus and bad bacteria jump on the opportunity to multiply.
- As the invaders rev up their engines, so do the cravings for refined carbs, sugar, chocolate, beer, wine, or hard liquor.
- If you feed these cravings — especially at night — you are literally feeding the bad microbes inside of your body.
- That's why even one glass of wine in the evening, which is seen by many as a harmless way to unwind, can make life very hard for the "good guys" battling it out in your gut.

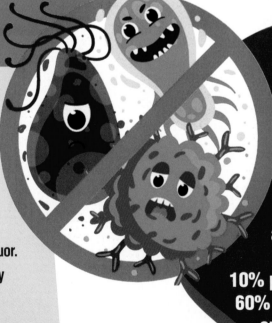

The average American eats 15 grams of fiber per day, instead of the 35 that they need for a healthy gut. In addition, the average American diet is 10% plant-based foods, 60% processed foods, and 30% animal products.

IMPORTANT JOBS THE GUT DOES

In the gut, the good bacteria:

- Identify the "bad guys" and usher them out of the system.
- Aid the body in the process of absorbing nutrients and turning them into energy.
- Work to keep the bad bacteria in the gut where it can be dealt with — and away from important body organs.

That's why much of the battle for your health — and to control your immune system — is won or lost in the gut.

How when you eat affects gut health:

- At night when you go to sleep your body enters into a rest, repair, and restore phase of healing.
- When your body and mind are in "shutdown mode," any extra energy is funneled to the biggest part of your immune system — the large intestine.
- As always, your "good guy" intestinal bacteria are standing guard, ready to attack and devour the vast quantities of parasitic microbes (such as "bad guy" bacteria and fungus) that come their way.
- If you eat before bedtime, and especially if what you eat is refined sugar or carbs, you have just been outsmarted by the bad bacteria living in your digestive tract.
- The vital energy that was needed to devour parasitic invaders must now be diverted to digest the food you just ate.

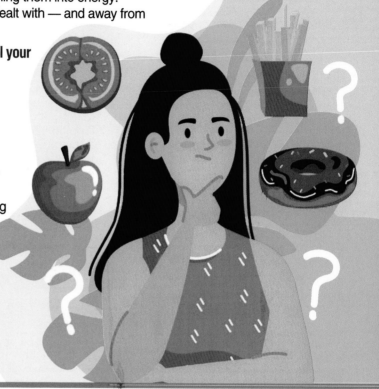

Your Ever-Evolving Gut

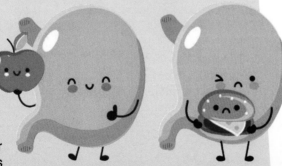

The microbes living in your gut aren't permanent residents. Like inhabitants of a thriving city, the "dwellers" in your microbial habitat come and go over time. Researchers have reported that a more diverse microbiome is a healthier microbiome. In other words, the more types of healthy gut bacteria operating within your system, the better. This diversity results in a more capable and resilient gut. The good news is we can control the kinds of bacteria that live in our gut. While some factors affecting our microbiome are hard if not impossible to change (e.g. genetics, illness, or stressful events), we can modify and control our diet and other lifestyle behaviors.

3 Foods Loved by "Bad" Gut Bacteria

1. **Highly processed foods and/or refined carbohydrates**
2. **Sugar (including artificial sweeteners)**
3. **Animal products**

Other Common Triggers for an Unhealthy Gut

- **Alcoholic beverages**
- **Antibiotics**
- **Certain medications**
- **High stress levels**
- **Irregularity in sleeping and eating**
- **Low fiber diet**
- **Sleep deprivation**

5 STRATEGIES FOR A HEALTHY GUT

1. **PLANT-BASED DIET:** High-fiber plant foods provide the best fuel for gut bacteria. A plant-based diet that includes a variety of fruit, legumes, vegetables, and whole grains increases the diversity of the gut microbiome, making it the very best diet for improving gut health.

2. **WHOLE FOODS:** Just because a diet is plant-based doesn't mean it is healthy. The key is to eat "whole" plant-based foods, which means to eat those foods in as much of a natural, unprepared state as possible. For a healthier gut, garden veggies are in and processed foods are out.

3. **DECREASE PESTICIDE EXPOSURE:** When shopping for any of the fruits or veggies known to be the most pesticide-laden (see the list of the "Dirty Dozen" on this page), try to look for organic, home grown, or chemical free. You may also try washing non-organic veggies with a baking soda rinse.

4. **HIGH FIBER FOODS:** While probiotics have received a lot of attention, fiber is really the "workhorse" iwn maintaining a healthy gut. High fiber foods, especially plant-based, are the menu of choice for good bacteria.

5. **DIETARY DIVERSITY:** Different bacteria — even the good ones — like different foods. So eat the rainbow! You can also mix things up by eating seasonally, avoiding dietary "ruts," and trying new things. Eating a diverse array of fruits and veggies is one of the best things you can do for your gut.

Dirty Dozen

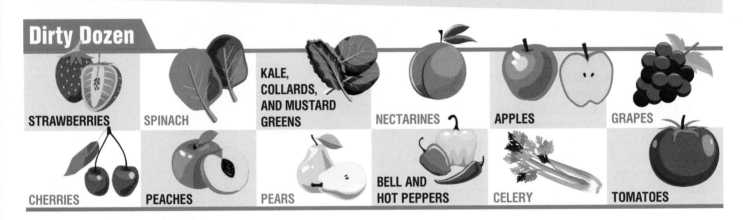

STRAWBERRIES

SPINACH

KALE, COLLARDS, AND MUSTARD GREENS

NECTARINES

APPLES

GRAPES

CHERRIES

PEACHES

PEARS

BELL AND HOT PEPPERS

CELERY

TOMATOES

SUPERFOODS THAT FEED HEALTHY GUT BACTERIA

These immune-boosting foods also raise metabolism, fight inflammation, and help to prevent colon cancer:

BANANAS: Fight inflammation, stabilize gut bacteria

BEANS: Boost satiety and absorption, release short-chain fatty acids

BLUEBERRIES: Enhance the immune system, destroy harmful bacteria

CRUCIFEROUS VEGGIES LIKE BROCCOLI: Sulfur-rich foods, fight inflammation and cancer

WHOLE GRAINS: Help to feed, grow, and sustain healthy gut bacteria

POLENTA: High in fiber, great-tasting

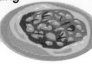

PLANT-BASED YOGURT: Improves health of intestinal tract, helps immune system function

TEMPEH: Crowds out bad bacteria, boosts nutrient absorption

Action Plan

→ Consider the health of your gut, and decide whether it can be improved or not.

→ Review this chapter, and make a list of diet changes you can make to improve gut health.

→ Plan how you can put those changes into action, and get started!

DIET NO-GO'S IN PANDEMIC TIMES
The Surprising Benefits of Giving Things Up

What Do "Pandemic Times" Have in Common with Lent, Ramadan, and Yom Kippur?

Every year, followers of certain faiths "give up" something as part of their religious practice:

- **During the month-long celebration of Lent every year, many Catholics give up "one thing."**
- **On Yom Kippur, the holiest day of the year for the Jewish faith, the devout abstain from food and drink for 24 hours.**
- **During the month-long Ramadan fast, Muslims don't eat, drink or engage in any sensual activity between sunrise and sunset.**

All this self-denial has opened the door for scientists to study the impact of "giving up" even just one thing on the immune system. As it turns out, making even one dietary change can pack a powerful immune-boosting punch. Which raises an important question: What if — just what if — giving up even one thing you normally do could provide a major boost to your health and longevity?

→ With so many people entertaining themselves in somewhat drastic ways (e.g. polar plunges!) during "Pandemic Times," what's so earth-shaking about pink-slipping a normally favorite food or drink? To the great benefit of your health, you could even take a "plunge" and delete a whole list of harmful foods. Difficult times call for stringent measures. Why not give your immune system every benefit possible in fighting off any virus that might come your way?

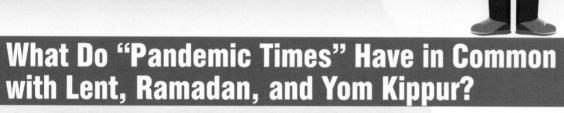

A little progress each day adds up to big results.

YOU ONLY GET ONE BODY, ONE TEMPLE TO TAKE CARE OF. IT'S OK TO START TODAY!

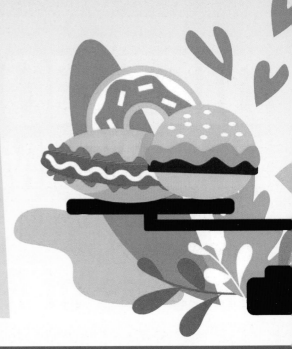

DIET NO-GO №1: Sugar

While sugar might seem like a comfort, it really is not your friend. Sugar does bad things to the body by:

- Lowering immune system function every single time it is eaten
- Reducing the ability of white blood cells to fight foreign bacteria
- Increasing inflammatory markers in the bloodstream
- Interfering with the body's transport of immune-boosting vitamin C
- Destroying good gut flora, which further depresses immune system function
- Leaching minerals from the body (giving it the unique ability to make people fat and malnourished at the same time)

TRY THIS: To satisfy a sweet tooth, eat some dates, honey, dried pineapple, or a touch of maple syrup.

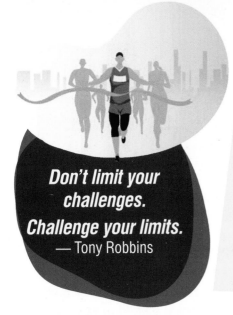

Don't limit your challenges.
Challenge your limits.
— Tony Robbins

Health Challenges Caused by Sugar

In addition to the above rap sheet of bad behavior, sugar consumption significantly increases the risk of a number of health challenges and diseases, including:

- Acne
- Alzheimer's Disease
- Cancer
- Cardiovascular disease
- Depression
- Diabetes
- Fatigue
- Headaches
- High blood pressure
- Hypertension
- Mental disorders
- Mood and behavioral problems
- Non-alcoholic Fatty Liver Disease (NAFLD)
- Obesity
- Tooth decay

To top it all off, sugar has virtually no nutritional value. That's why it's called "empty calories."

DIET NO-GO №2: White Flour (and other refined or processed foods)

White flour is harmful because it:
- Quickly converts to glucose in the body, thereby increasing sugar intake, which in turn weakens the immune system by reducing the number of white blood cells in the body
- Curbs the ability of the immune system to attack harmful bacteria
- Triggers blood sugar spikes and crashes, with the accompanying mood swings and energy drain

Like white flour, "enriched wheat flour" also signals that the package contents are a processed food. Processed foods:
- Fill the stomach with nutrient-poor, low-fiber foods
- Usually contain other harmful ingredients such as high fructose corn syrup, artificial ingredients, and trans fats
- Are generally high in salt

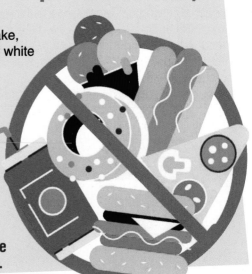

TRY THIS: Replace refined food choices with options that include whole flours or grains, and try making your own quick-and-easy healthier snacks.

DIET NO-GO №3: Excess Salt

Most people know that a salt-laden diet contributes to high blood pressure. Recent studies have shown that high salt intake is bad for the immune system as well. In one study, mice that were fed a high salt diet suffered from much more severe bacterial infections than mice who consumed less salt. In another study, human volunteers who ate an additional six grams of salt per day developed pronounced immune deficiencies. Cutting out fast foods and/or processed foods is the easiest way to drastically slash dietary salt intake. For those concerned about iodine, most processed foods do not contain iodized salt, so iodine needs to come from other sources anyway (preferably the iodized salt you use in cooking).

NOTE: While most people need to reduce salt intake, cutting out salt completely is not a good idea. An important nutrient, salt helps the body to balance fluids and maintain a healthy blood pressure.

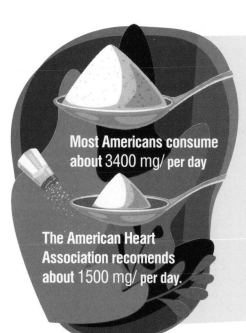

Most Americans consume about 3400 mg/ per day

The American Heart Association recomends about 1500 mg/ per day.

DIET NO-GO №4: Milk (and other dairy products)

Over the years, milk and dairy products have been lauded as important sources aof calcium and protein. In more recent times, dairy products have been closely linked to cancer and other health challenges. In one study, scientists from the University of California found that dairy products contain a molecule called Neu5Gc which isn't naturally produced by humans. Human cells react to Neu5Gc by producing antibodies against it. After years of consuming milk, this constant antibody production triggers a mild but continuous inflammatory response. Chronic inflammation, together with lowered immune system function, has long been linked to cancer. Other issues with milk are caused by casein, one of its primary proteins. In the human body, casein breaks down into a harmful compound known as beta casomorphin-7 (BCM7). In addition to affecting mood, this morphine-related compound causes cravings for dairy products. BCM7 has been linked to heart disease; it also has a negative health impact on the small intestines, hormonal function, and the immune system. In addition, milk products are mucus-forming for most people, which makes them more at risk for catching a cold or the flu.

TRY THIS: There are many delicious milk and even cheese substitutes available these days. The next time you are at the grocery store, try something new!

DIET NO-GO №5: Fried Foods

Fried food is especially bad for the immune system, for several reasons:

- Because of all the bad fats they contain, fried foods increase the cholesterol in our bodies, which in turn increases inflammation and decreases immune system function.
- Fried foods contain high levels of molecules known as advanced glycation end products (AGEs). AGEs are thought to weaken the immune system by depleting the body's antioxidant mechanisms, negatively affecting gut bacteria, promoting inflammation, and triggering cellular dysfunction. Researchers believe that diets high in AGEs may increase risk for certain cancers, heart disease, malaria, and metabolic syndrome.
- Fried foods contain acrylamide, which is believed to be, when eaten in sufficient quantities, a dangerous carcinogen.

TRY THIS: If you really like fried food, try baking instead of frying, or invest in an air fryer.

DIET NO-GO №6: Meat

Like fried foods, processed and charred meats are high in cancer-causing AGEs. Processed meats are also high in saturated fat, which contributes to systemic inflammation and reduced immune system function. A high intake of processed and charred meat has been linked to increased risk of colon cancer, among other diseases. As a high-acid food, meat of any type tips the body's pH in a less alkaline direction, which results in lower levels of minerals like magnesium, calcium, potassium and bicarbonate in the body. Barbecued or charred meats also contain significant levels of cancer-causing benzo(a)pyrene. These facts are just the tip of the "meatburg."

TRY THIS: Eat more legumes.

DIET NO-GO №8: Coffee

What does America's favorite morning brew have to do with immune system function? As it turns out, a lot. Coffee has been shown to:

- Trigger release of stress hormones (e.g. cortisol) that interfere with immune system function
- Block the production of infection fighting antibodies in the body
- Contribute to insomnia (which adds to immune system malfunction)

Coffee is also frequently accompanied by donuts, which, as mentioned in the "Diet No-Go" about sugar, lead to additional harmful effects.

TRY THIS: If you struggle to wake up, try a hot and cold shower! You could also try a coffee substitute or herbal teas.

DIET NO-GO №7: Alcohol

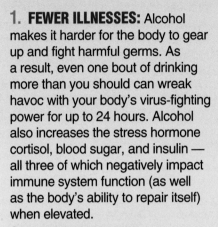

While society as a whole seems to think of alcohol as hard to give up, the truth is that substantial health benefits will be gained by abstention. Following is an overview of what to expect should you bid alcohol adieu:

1. **FEWER ILLNESSES:** Alcohol makes it harder for the body to gear up and fight harmful germs. As a result, even one bout of drinking more than you should can wreak havoc with your body's virus-fighting power for up to 24 hours. Alcohol also increases the stress hormone cortisol, blood sugar, and insulin — all three of which negatively impact immune system function (as well as the body's ability to repair itself) when elevated.

2. **A HEALTHIER LIVER:** Your liver's job is to filter toxins, including alcohol. Heavy drinking (which is defined as at least 15 weekly drinks for men and 8 or more for women) can take a toll on the organ, triggering fatty liver, cirrhosis, and other problems. The good news is that your liver can repair itself and regenerate within a matter of weeks. As a result, regular social drinkers who quit often see significant improvements in liver function in 30 days or less (heavy drinkers will take a bit longer).

3. **WEIGHT LOSS:** With a mostly empty calorie tally of 120-150 per glass, beer and wine significantly add to the beltline of many. Alcohol consumption also ramps up appetite and impulsivity, both of which make it harder to resist other menu temptations. Since obesity

contributes to lowered immunity, weight loss alone will be a boost to overall health.

4. **IMPROVED RELATIONSHIPS:** The lack of judgment that stems from even light alcohol use is the cause of many relationship problems. Alcoholism also decreases sex drive, adding even more fuel to the fire of already troubled relationships.

5. **LOWER BLOOD PRESSURE:** Alcohol use has been shown to contribute to higher blood pressure.

6. **REDUCED CANCER RISK:** Alcohol consumption has been linked to increased risk for several types of cancers, including cancers of the esophagus, mouth, throat, and breast.

7. **BETTER SLEEP:** Alcohol consumption disrupts the REM stage of sleep, wakes people up at night, and may even interfere with healthy breathing. For more restful shut-eye, abstinence is a great remedy.

8. **IMPROVED THINKING ABILITY:** Alcohol dependence can make it harder to think or remember things. It can also cloud perception of distances and volumes, impair motor skills, and make it harder to read the emotions of others.

TRY THIS: If you really want something carbonated, try some club soda!

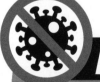

Action Plan

→ Review the "Diet No-Go's" described here and consider which of them you are currently eating and/or should give up.

→ Make a plan and take the (non-polar) plunge!

DRESS TO SUPPRESS
(Viruses, of Course)

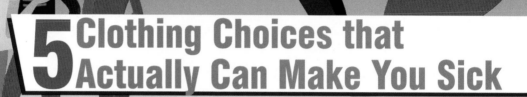

5 Clothing Choices that Actually Can Make You Sick

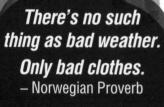

There's no such thing as bad weather.
Only bad clothes.
– Norwegian Proverb

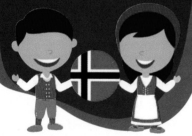

1 Inadequate Dress in Cold Weather

Although cold weather won't get you sick by itself, getting chilled can make it easier to catch a "bug." Researchers have found that exposure to cold temperatures can weaken the immune system, and thus the ability to fight infections.

2 Overdressing in Hot Weather

In hot weather, your body sweats as a way to cool down. If you are overdressed, you will dehydrate instead of cooling down. All that blood rerouting to your skin can strain other organs, thus lowering immune system function.

3 Wearing Tight Clothes

Tight jeans (or other tight-fitting clothes) can inhibit blood circulation, trigger swelling and numbness, and even cause muscle and nerve damage. For women, restrictive garments such as control-top hose and girdles can push on the organs, causing pain, acid reflux, and other serious digestive issues. Without good circulation, it's impossible for the immune system to perform at an optimal level.

4 Thin-soled Shoes on a Cold Floor

When one part of the body becomes cold, other parts of the body are affected as well. For example, when the feet become cold, the body reduces blood flow to the nose and throat. This protective measure, which is meant to keep blood flowing to the most vital organs, is called the "Reflex Effect." The reduced blood flow to the nose and throat leaves them devoid of the white blood cells, antibodies, and other protective substances normally relied on to fight off viruses and other invaders. The chain reaction between cold feet and catching a cold makes keeping the feet warm particularly important for immune system health.

5 Compression Pants or Leggings

Men and women who "hang out" in sweaty gym gear for too long after their workouts are at risk for a host of skin and bacterial conditions, including yeast infections. Compression workout tights made from nonbreathable fabric are most likely to create challenges. A shower and change of clothes shortly after any workout are recommended.

Keeping Your Core Just Right
Why Extremes of Heat and Cold Matter

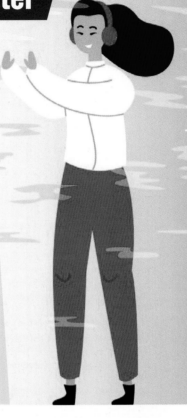

Although your body is set-up to handle fluctuations in surrounding temperatures, extreme heat — and cold — can overwhelm your internal temperature control system. Heat or cold stress, which happen when the body is unable to heat or cool itself properly, can weaken the immune system, leading to illness or even death.

COLD: If the body senses cold, it tries to protect its most important organs (brain, heart, and kidneys) by sending more blood in their direction. This leaves the hands, feet, and face with less blood circulation than they would have had. The lack of white blood cells and other resources in those areas makes it harder to heal quickly or fight off infections.

HEAT: When the surrounding environment is too hot, the internal thermostat of the body works to maintain a constant inner body temperature by pumping more blood to the skin, which results in sweat. The body uses sweat to increase the rate of heat loss. If the body becomes overwhelmed (e.g. the rate of heat gain exceeds the rate of heat loss), body temperature rises, leading to dehydration, heat stroke, or other heat-related illnesses.

BOTTOM LINE: When the body is kept from extremes of heat and cold, it doesn't have to work nearly as hard to maintain an optimal core temperature. A stable core temperature leaves more resources for fighting off outside invaders, which in turn leads to a stronger immune system.

PERFECT HEALTH REQUIRES PERFECT CIRCULATION.

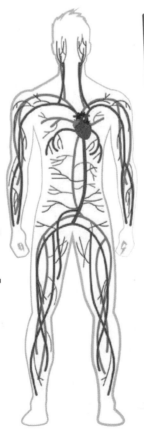

- **Tight-fitting clothes can impair circulation, thereby impairing health.**

- **Because the larger surface area of the body allows for more heat loss, tall people tend to become cold more easily than short individuals.**

RESEARCHERS HAVE DOCUMENTED THAT THE FOLLOWING ARE DECREASED THROUGH THE WEARING OF TIGHT CLOTHING:

- Bowel movement size
- Autonomic nervous system function
- Musculature activity of the trunk

At the same time, the following are increased:

- Digestive difficulties
- Back (lumbar) problems
- Length of time needed for passage of feces through the small intestine

Toxic Fabrics that May Harm Your Health

Not very long ago, people usually wore clothes made from natural fibers such as cotton, cashmere, hemp, linen, silk, and wool. In our modern world, clothing labels are much more likely to feature easy-to-wash, wrinkle-free fabrics that carry a chemical load most of us could do without. Following are five of the most toxic fabrics to watch out for:

POLYESTER: One of the most popular synthetic fabrics, polyester makes it harder for the skin to breathe. When the weather is hot and the skin is inhibited from breathing, body temperature may rise, prompting chemicals to be released from the fabric onto the skin. Dermatitis, eczema, itching, rashes, and redness are a few of the side effects that polyester can trigger.

RAYON: Toxic substances emitted by rayon fabric have been known to cause chest and muscle pain, headaches, insomnia, nausea, and/or vomiting.

NYLON: Clothing made from nylon fabric doesn't absorb sweat from the skin — an unfortunate feature that can lead to odors and/or skin infections. Bleach and dyes used in nylon can cause irritation as well.

ACRYLIC: The material used to make acrylic, acrylonitrile, is a known carcinogen and mutagen. Health problems that can be caused by acrylonitrile exposure include labored breathing, dizziness, headache, nausea, weakness of the limbs, and more.

SPANDEX: This popular stretchy fabric and those like it (e.g. Elastane, Lycra) are frequently used to make bikinis, leggings, sports bras, tights, and underwear. Unfortunately, they are made from harmful chemical substances (e.g. the carcinogen polyurethane). Skin irritations can be the result of prolonged exposure to these fabrics.

Keeping Germs Clear of Your Laundry
Researchers have found that:

- In addition to food and dirt from daily activities, laundry is a collector of waste from the human body.
- Blood, feces, saliva-born pathogens, and skin can all be transmitted by dirty laundry.
- When someone in a home is ill, the laundry may be contaminated and those doing the laundry exposed.
- Respiratory viruses (such as those that cause COVID-19) can last for a few days in the laundry, while diarrhea-causing viruses may last for a few weeks, and even grow, in the laundry.
- A normal wash cycle, together with effective laundry detergent, is sufficient to rid the laundry from bacteria, viruses, and other infectious agents.

What Shall I Wear?
The ideal clothing should be:

- Loose-fitting enough to allow good circulation
- Free of toxic chemicals
- Suitable to the climate and surrounding temperature
- Able to protect the body from heat and cold stress
- Of breathable fabric
- Regularly washed

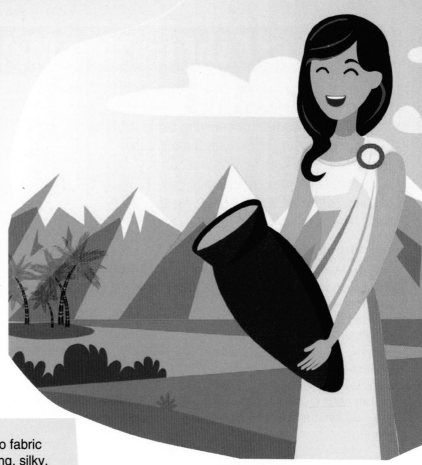

The Healthiest Fabrics to Wear

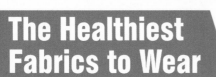

BAMBOO: A fascinating new option, bamboo fabric is breathable, hypoallergenic, thermo-regulating, silky, and soft. In addition to protecting from UV rays, bamboo fabric absorbs moisture from skin even better than cotton. It is also biodegradable.

CASHMERE: With its smooth and silky feel, cashmere is a natural fabric that feels amazing against the skin as well.

COTTON: This comfortable, time-honored fabric is breathable, durable, hypoallergenic, absorbs sweat well, and works with the body to protect against temperature changes.

HEMP: Known for its strength and durability, hemp has been a popular clothing fabric for thousands of years. This fabric, which holds its shape well, softens with use.

LINEN: This breathable, comfortable, and durable material is easy to care for and suitable for every season. It's also hypoallergenic.

MERINO WOOL: This lightweight, soft fabric is an all-natural, temperature and moisture regulating option that doesn't sag or lose shape over time. As an added bonus, it offers a natural UV protection. Alpaca wool is a similar alternative.

SILK: Renowned for its luxurious texture, silk clothing also packs a powerful health benefit punch, as researchers have found it to be anti-aging, anti-asthma, anti-eczema, and anti-fungal. Silk can also help to improve sleep.

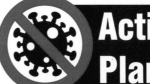

Action Plan

→ Consider whether any of your clothing choices are limiting the free circulation of blood, and if so, how you can change it.

→ Are you often chilled, or often overheated and sweating? If so, consider what you can do to relieve your body of cold or heat stress.

→ Consider the fabrics you are wearing. If you are already prone to eczemas or allergies, take a look at your wardrobe with an eye for how you could reduce the toxins faced by your body's largest organ.

Adopt a Chinchilla! NOT

Exotic pets are much more likely to carry disease than a dog or a cat.

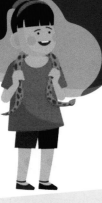

5 Important Things to Know About Exotic Pets

1 Exotic pets are very popular these days.

- In 2016, 13% of all U.S. households owned an exotic pet of some sort.
- 4.6% of all U.S. homes house a reptile as a pet.
- There are 5,000 privately held pet tigers in the U.S. alone.

2 The most popular exotic pets include...

- Amphibians (such as toads, salamanders, and frogs)
- Birds (including poultry)
- Fish, ferrets, and livestock
- Hamsters, guinea pigs, and gerbils
- Monkeys and rabbits
- Reptiles such as snakes, turtles, and lizards

3 Exotic pets carry many diseases.

- An estimated 90% of all reptiles are *Salmonella* carriers (e.g. iguanas, snakes, lizards, and turtles).
- Snakes carry two wormlike parasites, both of which can be transmitted to humans.
- Monkeys often carry the Herpes B virus or Monkeypox virus, both of which are dangerous when passed to humans.
- Virtually all exotic pets, including birds, rodents, fish, and primates, frequently carry diseases that can be deadly to humans.

4 Diseases that "jump" species from exotic pets to humans are the most dangerous.

Humans have co-existed with domesticated animals for centuries. As a result, the human immune system is much more prepared to ward off infection from commonly domesticated animals such as cats, dogs, horses, or cows. The same is not true for exotic or unusual pets, however. Diseases from these animals, when contracted, can make humans seriously ill.

5 Virus mutations are potentially lethal.

As viruses "copy themselves" within animals and humans, mistakes are made in the "copies." These mutations mean viruses are always changing — which makes them harder for the human immune system to recognize and ward off. The result of the ever-evolving viruses is extreme danger to humans. If a highly lethal virus jumps from an exotic animal to humans and mutates in a way that it becomes highly contagious, the results could be truly disastrous.

WHAT ARE ZOONOSIS
and why do they matter?

ZOONOSIS are diseases transmitted from animals to humans.

ZOO + NOSIS =
ANIMALS GIVING DISEASE

THEY COMPRISE:
- 60% of all infections in humans
- 75% of all emerging infectious diseases

5 Ways to "Catch" a Zoonotic Disease

1. Airborne transfer of viruses (e.g. if an animal sneezes or even breathes in your face)
2. Close proximity to animals (e.g. coming into contact with feces or fluids even if you did not touch the animal)
3. Direct contact through touching or bites
4. Through food
5. Vectors (e.g. bacteria and parasites passed from animals to humans)

Formula for a Pandemic

Trouble starts when a zoonotic disease jumps from an animal to a human. Then, if the virus:

- Mutates "successfully," enabling it to transmit from human to human,
- Is extremely contagious,
- Can travel by air (e.g. be passed by sneezes, coughs, or simply floating around), and
- Is terribly lethal, everything is "in order" for another terrible pandemic to start.

Some diseases currently plaguing the animal world are just a few mutations away from being transmitted to humans.

3 Facts to Know About Zoonotic Diseases

1. They leap from animals to humans and then (if they can) from human to human.
2. You don't have to eat an animal to get a zoonotic disease. Coming close to them — or a person who has, is dangerous enough.
3. They are, by far, the biggest health threat to the human race today.

How Scientists Can Trace the Source of Disease

- Throughout history, whenever a bad "bug" came along, humans were left wondering "where did this come from?"
- Questions about the origin of disease form the foundation of epidemiology, the branch of science which studies how diseases get started and spread.
- In the infancy of epidemiology, researchers tracked outbreaks by surveying people who had the disease.
- Through modern computer technology, researchers can now track an infectious disease across continents quickly and with amazing precision.
- Viruses and bacteria, which contain both DNA and RNA, are continually evolving and changing.
- As viruses copy themselves and spread, they make molecular mistakes (known as mutations).
- Although bacteria and viruses don't live very long, they replicate quickly in truly astonishing quantities. Because of this, changes in the virus can be seen within days or even just a few hours.
- Using advanced technology, researchers can now "sequence" infections from different people, observing how similar or dissimilar they are.
- When infections have a similar sequence, scientists know they came from the same part of the world.
- Although the work of tracking viruses can be very complicated, it can also be completed quickly and with remarkable accuracy with the aid of today's "super computers."

How a Little Wisconsin Girl Who Never Left Her Home State Got Monkeypox from a Rat in Gambia

1. Gambian Pouched Rats (exotic hamster-like pets which are now illegal in the United States) were imported by a Texas exotic animal importer.
2. The rats were shipped to Illinois, where an exotic animal distributor housed them with some prairie dogs.
3. The pouched rats, which were infected with Monkeypox, transmitted that disease to the prairie dogs.
4. The prairie dogs were shipped to Wisconsin, along with the disease.
5. A 3-year-old girl, who was bitten by a pet prairie dog, became hospitalized with symptoms which were eventually identified as Monkeypox.
6. All in all, 71 people across six Midwestern states were infected with Monkeypox.

This story had a happier ending than it might have. Although Monkeypox has a 10% fatality rate in Africa, no one died from this particular outbreak. Also, no human-to-human transmission was ever found. The incident does highlight, however, how an unexpected and unusual disease can get started based on infections, and choices, made far from the victims who eventually become ill.

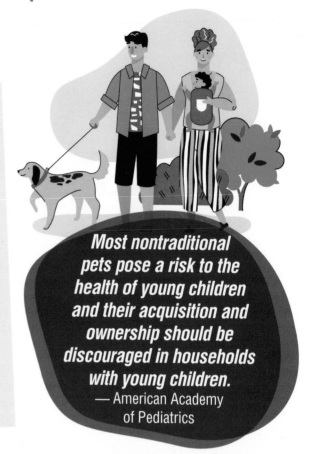

Most nontraditional pets pose a risk to the health of young children and their acquisition and ownership should be discouraged in households with young children.
— American Academy of Pediatrics

DEADLY ZOONOTIC DISEASES THROUGHOUT HISTORY

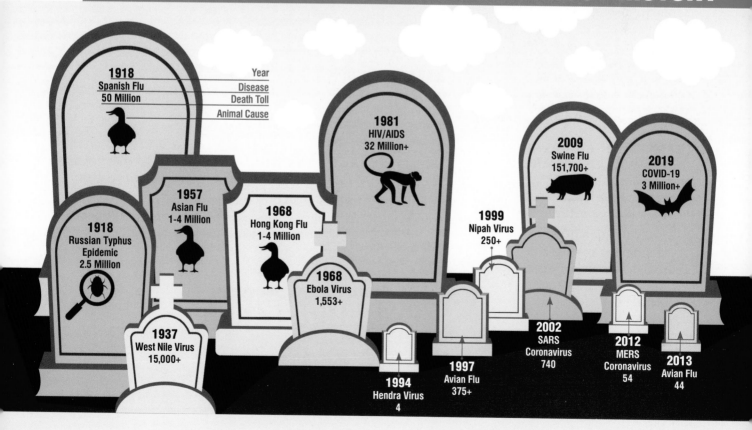

1918 Spanish Flu 50 Million

Year
Disease
Death Toll
Animal Cause

1918 Russian Typhus Epidemic 2.5 Million

1957 Asian Flu 1-4 Million

1968 Hong Kong Flu 1-4 Million

1981 HIV/AIDS 32 Million+

1968 Ebola Virus 1,553+

1937 West Nile Virus 15,000+

1994 Hendra Virus 4

1997 Avian Flu 375+

1999 Nipah Virus 250+

2002 SARS Coronavirus 740

2009 Swine Flu 151,700+

2019 COVID-19 3 Million+

2012 MERS Coronavirus 54

2013 Avian Flu 44

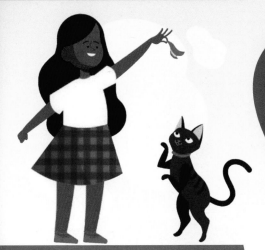

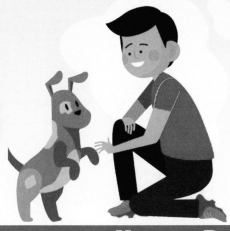

> If you would like to have a pet, the healthiest option would be a cat or a dog.

4 Health Benefits of Having a Cat

Owning a cat can be extremely rewarding. Feline friends love to have fun and play. They can also have a very calming effect on their owners. Following are some of the science-backed benefits of having a cat as a pet:

1. **LOWERED ANXIETY AND STRESS:** Researchers have found that a cat's purr can not only calm the nervous system, but lower blood pressure as well. And, as any cat owner can confirm, one good session of play can make a bad day into a better one.

2. **IMPROVED CARDIOVASCULAR HEALTH:** Scientists have reported that cat owners have a reduced risk for heart disease and/or stroke.

3. **ALLERGY PREVENTION:** Children who are exposed to cats within the first few years of life are more likely to develop an immune system that combats allergies effectively.

4. **REDUCED LONELINESS:** With their unconditional love and purring affection, cats make a great companion for lonely hearts.

8 Reasons to Have a Dog

Researchers have found that spending time with a pup can do wonders for your well-being — both physically and emotionally. Following are 10 evidence-based benefits of having a four-footed canine best friend:

1. **COMPANIONSHIP:** When other people can't be there for us (e.g. social isolation), dogs make us feel less alone.

2. **IMPROVED CARDIOVASCULAR HEALTH:** Dog owners tend to have lower blood pressure, improved heart health, and a lower overall risk of death.

3. **REDUCED ANXIETY AND STRESS:** Even just petting a dog has been shown to lower blood pressure, slow breathing, reduce cortisol (a major stress hormone), and relax muscle tension.

4. **BETTER COPING SKILLS:** Military veterans with a service dog have been found to have less PTSD and better coping skills overall.

5. **A MORE ACTIVE LIFE:** Researchers have found that, with an average of 300 minutes weekly walking their dogs, dog owners are four times more active than non-dog owners.

6. **MORE SOCIAL OPPORTUNITIES:** Walking your dog is more than exercise — it's also a perfect way to make new friends. Researchers have found that people with a strong attachment to a pet feel more connected in their human relationships and their communities.

7. **A HIGHER HAPPINESS QUOTIENT:** Japanese researchers found that just staring into a dog's eyes raises levels of oxytocin, also known as the "love hormone." Those little tail-waggers are natural mood boosters!

8. **IMPROVED THINKING ABILITY:** Pet therapy has been shown to improve cognitive function, reduce agitation, and lead to more positive social interactions for seniors in long-term care.

Action Plan

→ Consider your exposure to exotic pets, and the health dangers it may entail. Think about ways to reduce or eliminate that exposure, and put your plan into action.

→ If you would like a companion pet, consider a cat or a dog.

EAT, DRINK & BE STRONG:
Let These Foods Dominate Your Plate

Let food be your medicine, and medicine be your food.
— Hippocrates

The Insulin Impact

Insulin resistance is a huge problem in the United States, where 60-70 million individuals suffer from the malady (with many more being at risk). Insulin resistance impacts the immune system in very significant ways, which is why so many diabetics have struggled against COVID-19. Following are some important things to know about the impact of diet on this key health challenge:

- When a person who is insulin resistant eats, fasting glucose starts to go up above normal levels.
- The excess glucose begins sticking to the white blood cells, which in turn impairs immune system function.
- Studies have shown that the more sugar you eat, the less effectively your immune system works.
- Although sugar is bad for you, the №1 enemy in insulin resistance is fat. Diets high in saturated fat (such as is found in meat, dairy, and eggs) have been found to increase insulin resistance.
- The best diet to decrease insulin resistance is a whole foods, plant-based diet.

THE FOOD-IMMUNE SYSTEM CONNECTION

Nitric Oxide: What You Should Know, and Why

Hailed as the "miracle molecule," nitric oxide is a powerful blood circulation optimizer that is vital to the health of virtually every cell, organ, and system in the body — including the immune system.

- The body produces its own nitric oxide. However, production decreases as we age. By age 70, humans have lost 70% of their ability to generate nitric oxide.
- The ability to generate nitric oxide can be restored with a diet rich in natural nitrates.
- Nitric oxide specializes in vasodilation, a process which relaxes and widens the inner blood vessels, resulting in increased circulation and lower blood pressure.
- Because of the powerful positive effect it has on the body, nitric oxide is a vital first line of defense against viral infections.
- Added nitrates, such as those in bacon, deli meat, hot dogs, and ham, have been strongly linked to cancer, among other health challenges. They are not a good source for this valuable nutrient.

In recent research, nitric oxide has been shown to prevent the replication of coronaviruses.

Foods Rich in Natural Nitrates

| Leafy Greens | Garlic | Nuts | Seeds |

G-BOMBS®

| Greens | Beans | Onions | Mushrooms | Berries | Seeds |

- One of the best ways to remember the healthiest foods to eat is by using the "G-BOMBS®" acronym coined by Dr. Joel Furhmann.

- These nutrient-rich, cancer-fighting foods, which are extremely protective against chronic disease, are the best foods on the planet for promoting health and longevity.

- They are also the very best food choices to aid the body in building a stronger immune system.

G is for Greens

Packed with nutrients and phytochemicals, leafy greens are some of the healthiest foods on the planet. These life-giving veggies get their vibrant color from chlorophyll, a nutrient-rich green substance that carries with it a host of benefits to the human body. The abundance of oxygen and healthy blood flow promoted by chlorophyll encourages the removal of harmful impurities and toxins, strengthens the immune system, and helps put the body into a more alkaline state. Following is an overview of health benefits associated with specific greens within this incredible group of superfoods:

ARUGULA: Slows down cancer growth, improves immune system function, promotes the growth of healthy bones.

COLLARD GREENS: Boost immune system in the fight against viral and bacterial infections, help lower LDL cholesterol, regulate blood sugar, combat osteoporosis.

ICEBERG LETTUCE: Combats anemia, age-related illnesses, and heart disease.

KALE: Aids in blood clotting, promotes better vision, fights cancer.

MUSTARD GREENS: Protect against anemia, arthritis, cancer, and cardiovascular disease.

ROMAINE LETTUCE: Prevents cancer and strokes. Promotes heart health and healthier bones, eyes, skin, and mucous membranes.

SPINACH: Improves red blood cell function, strengthens bones, regulates blood pressure and heart rate, combats free radicals.

SWISS CHARD: Regulates heart rate, blood pressure, and blood sugar levels. Prevents anemia, boosts immunity, and helps maintain connective tissues.

TURNIP GREENS: Boost immune defenses against cancer and other illnesses. Enhance collagen synthesis, build healthy bones, and combat anemia.

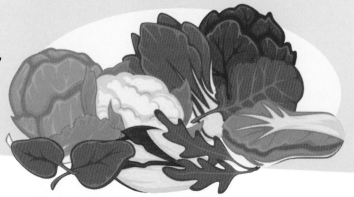

B is for Beans

A nutritional powerhouse, beans are:

RICH IN PROTEIN: Which plays an important role in building immune system cells. As an added benefit, they are lower in calories and saturated fat than other protein sources (e.g. meat, eggs, and dairy products).

AN EXCELLENT SOURCE OF FOLATE: A B vitamin and important immune system booster.

HIGH IN FIBER: Which makes them very beneficial in the fight against invading viruses and pathogens.

RICH IN POLYPHENOLS: Antioxidants which protect the body from disease by helping it to remove damaging chemicals known as free radicals.

EXCELLENT FOR THE HEART: Researchers have found a clear correlation between eating beans and reduced risk of cardiovascular disease. Beans have also been shown to help lower cholesterol — another heart-related health benefit.

PROTECTIVE AGAINST CANCER: Due to their anti-oxidant and anti-inflammatory properties.

STABILIZERS OF BLOOD GLUCOSE LEVELS: The high fiber content of beans helps them to lower and/or stabilize blood glucose levels, which in turn helps lower the risk for Type 2 Diabetes.

GOOD FOR THE LIVER: Replacing high fat animal proteins with beans is an important step towards addressing fatty liver disease, as well as achieving better overall health.

HELPFUL FOR APPETITE CONTROL: The fiber and helpful starches contained in beans help create the full and satisfied feeling which makes it easier to push the plate away.

BENEFICIAL FOR THE GUT: Researchers have found that a variety of beans in the diet feed and boost the beneficial bacteria in the gut, which is a critical component of immune system function.

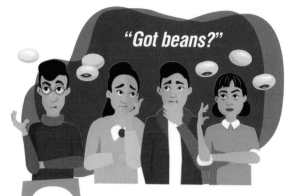

"Got beans?"

O is for Onions

Although "onions" make up the "O" in the G-Bombs acronym, this category includes the entire Allium plant family. Rich in vitamins, minerals, and other health-promoting compounds, onions and their Allium cousins are very beneficial to both the immune system and overall health. Healthful compounds contained in this wonderful group of veggies include:

ANTIOXIDANTS: Researchers have found a strong link between antioxidant-rich diets and reduced cancer risk. Antioxidant rich foods have also been linked to improved immune system function.

FLAVONOIDS: Chives, garlic, onions, and leeks all contain flavonoids which promote the production of glutathione, a powerful antioxidant which has been shown to boost the immune system, help detox the body, and protect the heart. Virtually every cell in your body needs glutathione, which is why it has been nicknamed "the mother of all antioxidants."

BENEFITS TO BE DERIVED FROM EATING ALLIUM VEGGIES INCLUDE:

- Improved cardiovascular health, including lower triglycerides, increased HDL cholesterol, reduced blood pressure, and protection against plaque buildup.
- Reduced risk of blood clots.
- Antimicrobial protection against *E. coli*, viruses, *Staphylococcus aureus*, oral bacteria, and parasites.
- An anti-inflammatory effect, which can be particularly helpful in cases of arthritis and/or painful joints and is helpful for health overall.

Members of the Allium family

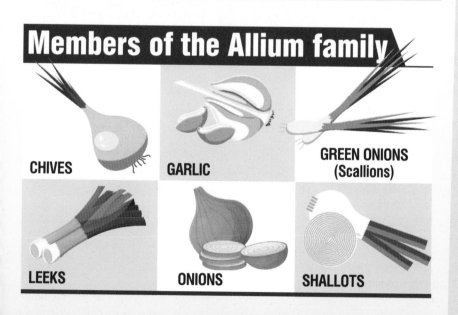

CHIVES

GARLIC

GREEN ONIONS (Scallions)

LEEKS

ONIONS

SHALLOTS

CHAPTER 11

M is for Mushrooms

What marvelous mushrooms can do for you:

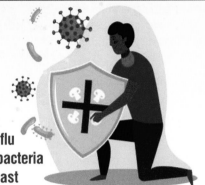

- Boost your immune system
- Destroy cancer cells
- Facilitate nerve regeneration
- Provide valuable nutrients
- Help with weight management
- Eradicate viruses (including the flu and pox viruses like smallpox), bacteria (*Salmonella* and *E. coli*), and yeast

S is for Seeds (and Nuts)

Because seeds contain all the necessary nutrients to develop an entire plant, they are extremely nutritious. Packed with fiber, seeds are also loaded with healthy fats — not to mention antioxidants, vitamins, and minerals. Following is an overview of some of the most helpful seeds you can eat:

PUMPKIN SEEDS: The most alkaline-forming seed, these little nutritional powerhouses come stocked with heart-healthy magnesium, zinc for immune support, plant-based omega-3 fats, and vitamins B, K, and E.

SUNFLOWER SEEDS: While the vitamin E in these seeds helps to neutralize free radicals, phytosterols help lower cholesterol, and magnesium protects against migraines and heart disease.

SESAME SEEDS: These tiny seeds contain compounds that help to reduce stress, relieve tension, fight arthritis, protect against cancer, and promote respiratory health.

FLAX SEEDS: High in antioxidants and omega-3 fats, flax seeds are also great for improving digestion and cardiovascular health.

HEMP SEEDS: Hemp seeds are loaded with vitamins A, B1, B2, D, and E. The zinc in hemp seeds supports oxygen production, healthy digestion, blood sugar stabilization, and lower cholesterol levels.

THE SKINNY ON NUTS

As for nuts, the superstars in this category (such as almonds and walnuts) contain the vitamin E needed by the immune system to ward off invading bacteria plus the healthy fat needed to absorb it. Many studies have shown that those who eat nuts on a regular basis have longer and healthier lives.

NOTE: Nuts and seeds are healthiest raw and unsalted.

B is for Berries

Small in size but giant in nutritional value, berries are one of the healthiest foods you can eat. Berries are literally packed with vitamins, minerals, and antioxidants which are extremely important to immune system function. Berries are one of nature's best sources of antioxidants — especially the three listed below:

ANTHOCYANINS
- Regulate immune response
- Calm inflammation
- Enhance memory
- Protect against cardiovascular disease

QUERCETIN
- Stimulates the immune system
- Fights viruses
- Inhibits histamine release
- Fights inflammation

VITAMIN C
- Boosts white blood cell production
- Enhances overall immune system function
- Protects memory and thinking ability
- Lowers risk of cardiovascular disease

In addition to these benefits, berries are low in calories (making them great for weight management).

Action Plan

Take a look at your normal daily diet, and consider it in light of the information in this chapter. Ask yourself the following questions, then, if need be, make and put into action a plan to improve:

→ Am I getting enough nitric oxide in my diet from natural sources?

→ Do the foods I eat help to keep my blood sugar levels stable?

→ Which of the G-BOMB® food categories do I regularly eat?

→ How can I improve my diet?

LET THE SUN SHINE IN:
For a Health-promoting Win

Sunshine kills germs…

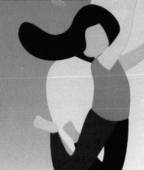

…and it doesn't like COVID, either.

6 Ways Sunshine Boosts the Immune System

1 Sunshine is a Disinfectant

For some time, people have understood what your grandma knew decades ago: sunlight kills germs. In an Oregon study, researchers found that sunlit rooms had half the germs of their darkened counterparts, proving once again that sunlight is a powerful disinfectant.

2 Sunshine Helps the Body Make Vitamin D

At any given time, about 40% of Americans are said to be low on vitamin D. This is especially dangerous during these virus-laden times, since vitamin D is so important to healthy immune system function. Sunlight is an inexpensive, quick, and painless way to boost levels of this valuable and extremely necessary vitamin.

3 Sunlight Stimulates Melatonin Production

Since melatonin regulates when your immune system is activated, getting enough sunshine — and melatonin — is a pretty big deal! Melatonin can also reduce both chronic and acute inflammation.

4 Sunlight Reduces Stress

Scientists believe that sunlight boosts mood by releasing serotonin, a feel-good hormone. Sunlight's creation of melatonin also triggers a stress reducing effect on the body.

5 Sunlight Energizes Infection-fighting T Cells

In recent research, scientists found that sunlight energizes the body's T cells, which in turn play a central role in human immunity. This function is separate — and in addition to — the sun's very beneficial role in vitamin D production.

6 Sunlight Aids in the Absorption of Immune-boosting Minerals such as Calcium and Phosphorous

Sunlight serves as the primary source of vitamin D for most people. It also plays a direct role in the body's absorption of calcium, which is needed to produce melatonin. Without adequate sunlight, many people don't have enough vitamin D in their bodies to help process the calcium they so badly need. Although vitamin D's most dramatic effect is facilitating calcium intake, it also stimulates the absorption of the much-needed phosphate and magnesium ions as well.

May you always walk in the sunshine. May you never want for more.
— Irish Blessing

Colors of Light and Their Healing Effect

When you pull back the curtains and sunshine floods into the room, that "white" light which brightens your spirits is known as "full spectrum" light. Calling a light "full spectrum" means that it covers the entire range of wavelengths needed by animals and plants. Although lighting manufacturers label some indoor lighting as "full spectrum," there is nothing quite like the sun for blanketing a room with brilliance! When all the colors of the spectrum are combined together, the result is the nearly blinding "white" or bright light that we experience under the bright rays of the sun.

The various colors of light in the spectrum have different electromagnetic wavelengths. Some of those wavelengths penetrate more deeply into the human body than others, and each wavelength has its own healing properties.

In recent years, inventors have become increasingly adept at isolating certain wavelengths (colors) of light. Soaking in the rays of the sun outdoors is the best way to benefit from the entire healing spectrum. However, if you aren't able to get out much, or need a concentrated wavelength for a specific health purpose, there are now scientifically-backed therapy lights on the market which will deliver just that. Following is an overview of the light spectrum, with some of the proven healing benefits for each color / wavelength in the spectrum.

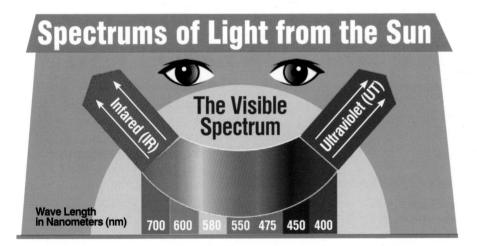

Spectrums of Light from the Sun

Infared (IR)

The Visible Spectrum

Ultraviolet (UT)

Wave Length in Nanometers (nm): 700 600 580 550 475 450 400

Benefits of Red and Infrared Light

- Nitric oxide production
- Increased circulation
- Collagen production
- Faster wound healing
- Better nerve function
- Anti-viral properties
- ATP (raw cellular energy) production
- Lymphatic stimulation
- Reduced inflammation

Benefits of Ultraviolet (UV) Light

- Interacts with the skin to produce vitamin D
- Aids the immune system
- Reduces the risk of disease
- Promotes longevity

NOTE: Depending on type, ultraviolet light penetrates between 5 and 3 mm into the skin. Excess UV light can cause cancer.

Benefits of Orange Light

Orange light therapy results in many of the same benefits as red. They just take longer, as the treatment is not as intense.

Uses of Amber Light

When placed over blue light, amber filters alter its melatonin-restricting properties and allows the brain to transition to sleep. This is why many blue-blocking filters are amber or orange, which, like red, are considered good for melatonin production and sleep in general.

Benefits of Green Light

Green light is helpful for:

- Migraine relief
- Pain reduction
- Better comprehension

Benefits of Blue Light

- Highly anti-bacterial
- Calms the nervous system
- Energizes the brain
- Elevates mood
- Tells the brain it is daylight (when perceived by the eyes)
- Assists hormones and transmitters that impact appetite, metabolism, and sleeping

Blue Light in the Morning is Wonderful; Blue Light at Night, Not So Much

How night time blue light affects your body and brain

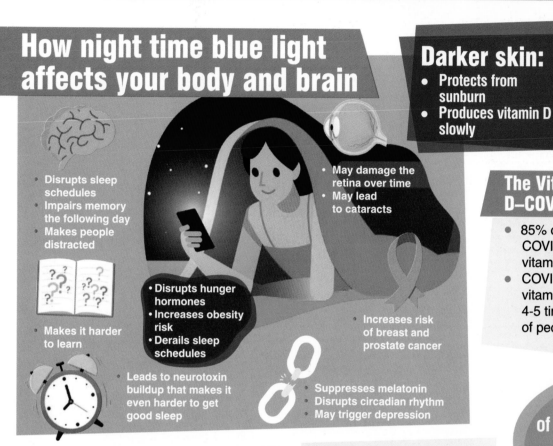

- Disrupts sleep schedules
- Impairs memory the following day
- Makes people distracted
- Makes it harder to learn

- Disrupts hunger hormones
- Increases obesity risk
- Derails sleep schedules

- Leads to neurotoxin buildup that makes it even harder to get good sleep

- May damage the retina over time
- May lead to cataracts

- Increases risk of breast and prostate cancer

- Suppresses melatonin
- Disrupts circadian rhythm
- May trigger depression

Darker skin:
- Protects from sunburn
- Produces vitamin D slowly

Lighter skin:
- Burns easily in the sun
- Produces vitamin D quickly

The Vitamin D–COVID Connection

- 85% of people with severe COVID-19 were found to have vitamin D deficiency.
- COVID-19 sufferers with vitamin D deficiency had 4-5 times the mortality rate of people with normal levels.

81% of African Americans and 69% of Hispanics are deficient in vitamin D.

The Vitamin D — Sunshine Connection

Although the sun confers many health benefits, one of the most vital (and well known) is the production of vitamin D. Following are some key facts you should know about this important vitamin:

- Vitamin D is an essential fat-soluble vitamin that acts much like a hormone in the body.
- Maintaining a sufficient level of vitamin D is important for all aspects of health.
- About a third of the world's population is deficient in vitamin D.
- Adults with a vitamin D deficiency have an increased risk of death from heart disease (35%), cancer (14%), twice the risk of developing osteoarthritis, a 51% higher chance of developing dementia, and a heightened overall mortality risk.

Most of Our Vitamin D Comes from the Sun

- Exposure of arms and legs for 5-30 minutes between the hours of 10 a.m. and 3 p.m. two days per week can be enough to prevent deficiency.
- Sunlight is strong enough to produce vitamin D whenever your shadow is shorter than you.
- In the winter, the sun isn't intense enough to provide the needed vitamin D (especially in northern climates).
- Sunscreen, clothing, and glass all reduce vitamin D absorption.

Plant-based Ways to Get Vitamin D

- Mushrooms exposed to UV light
- Vitamin D-enriched foods
- Vitamin D3 supplements

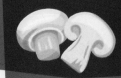
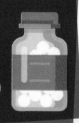

BENEFITS OF VITAMIN D

The Sunshine Vitamin

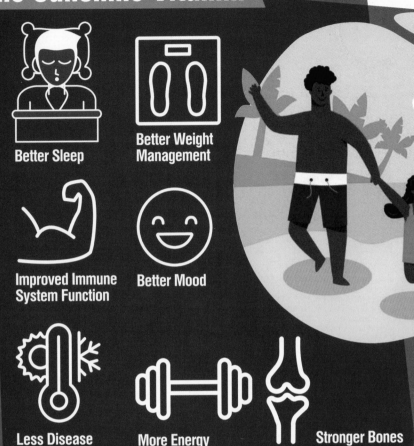

Better Sleep

Better Weight Management

Improved Immune System Function

Better Mood

Less Disease

More Energy

Stronger Bones

Action Plan

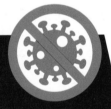

→ Consider whether you are getting enough sunlight in your life. If not, make a plan to get out and catch some rays!

→ Think about your nighttime routine. Are you using blue screen technology until just before going to bed? If so, consider the health consequences and what you could do to improve.

→ If you've never had your vitamin D checked, or haven't had it checked lately, consider that now might be a good time. If you find that you aren't able to get enough vitamin D either through sunlight exposure or diet, you might want to check into supplementation.

How Sunshine and Exercise are Alike

If you aren't able to hike or bike like you used to, or simply want to do two health-promoting activities at once, you may be happy to know that sunshine and exercise do some of the very same things. Here's an overview of benefits exercise and sun bathing share:

Both Decrease:
- Blood sugar levels
- Lactic acid in the blood
- Resting heart rate
- Respiratory rate

Both Increase:
- Basal rate of metabolism
- Energy and endurance
- Hormone production
- Strength
- Stress tolerance

TAKEWAY: If you're feeling like a "couch tater," why not at least turn into a "sun tater" instead?

MOVE MORE, SIT LESS:

Why Sitting is the New Smoking

Sitting: The new national pastime!

IN THE UNITED STATES:

- 80% of jobs require no physical activity
- Office workers sit for an average of 12 hours per day
- The "average Joe" sits for 9.3 hours per day

Sitting is an independent risk factor for a weak immune system. HERE'S WHY:

When you sit for 30 minutes:
- The body becomes less sensitive to insulin.
- Electrical activity and muscles in the lower body and legs are turned off.
- Enzymes that move the bad fat from the arteries to the muscles, where it can get burned off, slow down.
- Brain activity starts to decrease.
- Metabolism drops by up to 90%.
- Calorie-burning activity plummets.

When you sit for 2 hours:
- Breakdown of dangerous blood fats becomes slower.
- HDL ("good") cholesterol drops by 20%.

When you sit for 4 hours:
- Risk of death from any cause rises by 50%.
- Risk of a cardiovascular event skyrockets by up to 125%.

When you sit for 6 hours:
- Oxygen consumption levels decrease, making even simple exercises more difficult.
- Risk of colon cancer rises by 2X.
- Risk of rectal cancer rises by 44%.

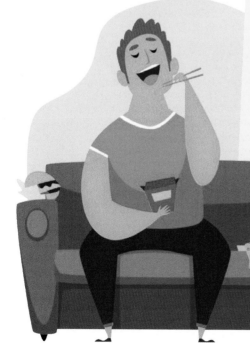

Sitting is more dangerous than smoking, kills more people than HIV, and is more treacherous than parachuting. We are sitting ourselves to death. The chair is out to kill us.
— Dr. James Levine, Mayo Clinic

The High Cost of "Sitting Around"

- Today's sedentary lifestyle has been linked to more than 30 chronic health conditions, not to mention skyrocketing healthcare costs.
- In one 2008 study, researchers found inactivity to be the causal factor in 9% of the world's premature deaths.
- The adipose tissues of the body (fat) produce pro-inflammatory cytokines.

The Obesity — COVID-19 Connection

When we don't move, our inactivity leads to abdominal fat. As a result of this, some normally "good guy" cell sentinels in the body known as macrophages infiltrate the fat cells, triggering chronic inflammation, which eventually leads to disease. When COVID-19 strikes, a similar process takes place. To try to fight off the infection, the immune system sentinel cells overreact by "calling in" too many troops. This overreaction results in the very dangerous cytokine storm where, in an effort to defeat the virus, the body attacks its own organs. The result is tissue damage in various organs, especially the lungs. This explains why the following equation is so tragically true:

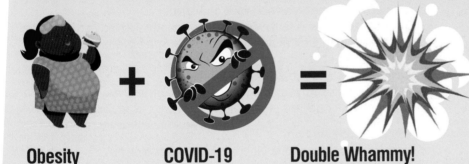

Obesity + **COVID-19** = **Double Whammy!**

The Dangerous Cluster of Disease Related to Sitting:

- Breast Cancer
- Colon Cancer
- Cardiovascular Diseases
- Diabetes
- Depression
- Dementia

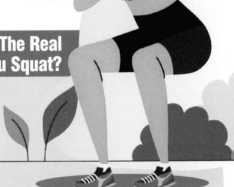

NEWS FLASH!

1. Researchers have found that getting active is one of the fastest ways to improve your health.

2. Being active at least 7 hours per week reduces your chance of dying early by 40% over those who are only active 30 minutes per week.

Time to get moving!

Forget Sitting vs Standing: The Real Question Should Be, Should You Squat?

- For most of human history, the "squat" has been the preferred form of resting.
- In most of the "Blue Zones" (areas of the world where people live the longest), more people squat than not.
- In many areas of the world, people squat to milk cows, harvest seaweed, tend to rice, or to relieve themselves.
- Squatting utilizes more core muscles than either sitting or standing. Perhaps that's why the ability to squat translates into healthy hips, a healthier spine, and a lower risk of dying in the next 6 years.
- The ability to easily rise from either a squatting position or sitting on the floor (while touching as few body parts to the ground as possible) has been found to be a predictor of how soon you could die.

BENEFITS OF EXERCISE

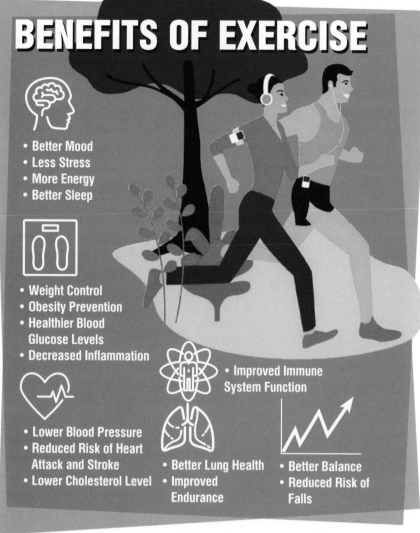

- Better Mood
- Less Stress
- More Energy
- Better Sleep

- Weight Control
- Obesity Prevention
- Healthier Blood Glucose Levels
- Decreased Inflammation

- Lower Blood Pressure
- Reduced Risk of Heart Attack and Stroke
- Lower Cholesterol Level

- Improved Immune System Function

- Better Lung Health
- Improved Endurance

- Better Balance
- Reduced Risk of Falls

What Makes Sustained Physical Exercise So Powerful

- Engaging in sustained physical exercise is one way of creating an artificial fever. During a long and intense exercise session, the body temperature can climb as high as 104°F (40°C).
- As body temperature rises, oxygen and energy flood the cells and burn away body wastes. Toxins that are embedded in the tissues are dismantled, all the way down to the cellular level.
- For those with the strength and endurance to do it, 1-2 hours of hearty regular exercise will contribute greatly to restoring the integrity of the internal cellular environment and overall health.

Effect of Exercise on Immune System Function

RISK of Upper Respiratory Tract Infections

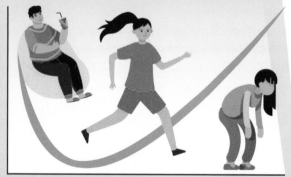

Sedentary   Moderate   Overtraining
EXERCISE

TAKEAWAYS FROM THE CHART ABOVE:

1. Being a couch potato reduces immune system function and increases risk of diseases.
2. Moderate exercise boosts immune system function.
3. Overtraining, especially when sick, drains vital energy needed by the immune system to fight off "bugs."

SCORECARD
Pharmaceuticals vs Exercise

PHARMACEUTICALS
- An estimated 328,000 people die from adverse reactions to prescription drugs each year in the U.S. and Europe combined.
- Approximately 7,000 patients die each year from being given the wrong medication.
- About 80,000 die each year from infections contracted at the facility of their medical care provider.

EXERCISE
- Exercise-related heart attacks are quite rare, accounting for just 5% of cardiac arrests.
- Regular exercise has been shown to improve heart function and slow disease progression in patients with heart disease.
- A 12-month exercise program for stable heart patients was found to be superior to angioplasty as a treatment.

WALKING: One of the Very Best Exercises to Improve Physical Fitness

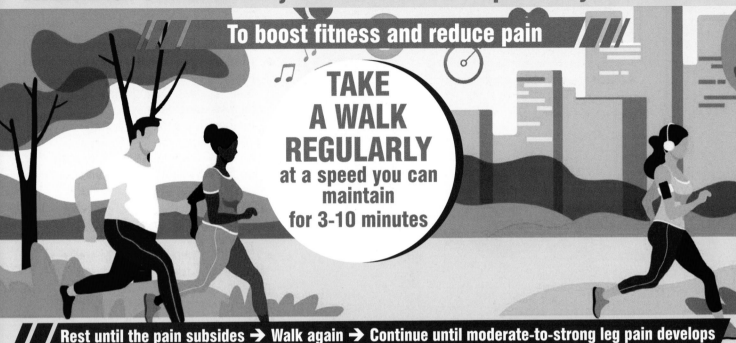

To boost fitness and reduce pain

TAKE A WALK REGULARLY at a speed you can maintain for 3-10 minutes

Rest until the pain subsides → Walk again → Continue until moderate-to-strong leg pain develops

Interval Training for Walkers: A 10-Step Program

1. Wear comfortable clothing.
2. Stay hydrated.
3. Choose walking routes with resting places.
4. Find a walking partner.
5. Follow the walk-rest-walk suggestion in the illustration above, starting with whatever length of time you think you can handle.
6. Build up your walking speed and length of walks over time.
7. Avoid sidewalks if you have joint pain. Walking on trails and grass creates less impact on your joints.
8. Don't walk if you feel unwell.
9. If you experience chest pain, dizziness, or other illness, seek medical advice.
10. Be patient! It usually takes several weeks for signs of improvement to appear.

WALKING PROMOTES:

- Better sleep
- Concentration
- Energy levels
- Cardiovascular health
- Joint & muscle health
- Weight management
- Lung health
- Stress relief

THE 4 PARTS OF AN EXERCISE PROGRAM

F = Frequency (how often?)

I = Intensity (how hard?)

T = Time (how long?)

T = Type (what kind?)

Action Plan

→ Consider how much time you spend sitting each day. If it's too much, what could you do to improve?

→ If you're physically able, try squatting. Think about how you could add a bit of squatting into your daily routine.

→ If you are able to walk at all, get started with a daily walking program, even if that means only walking across the room a few times to start. Use the FITT prescription to set-up your plan.

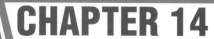

CRY FOWL:
Chicken Soup is Not Good for Your Soul

Where chicken soup used to cure you from the flu, now it gives you the flu.

— Jay Leno

THE CHICKEN WITHIN THE SOUP:
From the Factory to Your Table

The vast majority of chickens being eaten in soup or in other forms today were raised on factory farms. Here's what you should know about them:

- Chicken-to-chicken spread of disease on factory farms causes viruses to adapt quickly into even more dangerous strains. As a result, world health organizations have come to view factory farms as virtual "incubators" for emergent diseases.
- Even the poultry industry is beginning to recognize that viruses which were relatively harmless to their original host species have become deadlier with each pass through commercial farms.
- Viruses are brought into and out of farms by rodents and other pests, which pass them back and forth to migrating birds, which then "fly" them between countries.
- The first human cases of the latest avian flu virus, H5N8, were reported by the Russian Federation in February of 2021. Although the first humans have been asymptomatic, health authorities the world over are deeply concerned that some form of an avian flu will mutate into a highly lethal virus that's easily passed between humans.
- Multiple countries are reporting that the "culling" (elimination) of literally millions of birds has not effectively stopped the "Bird Flu," which continues to mutate and spread.

8 Fast Facts About Chicken

1. During the 1800's, chicken was considered to be a food for the rich.
2. Eating chicken didn't increase in popularity until the World War II pork and beef shortages.
3. U.S. chicken consumption really took off in the 1990's when doctors started suggesting less red meat and people began fearing Mad Cow Disease.
4. Today, chicken is the most popular protein in the United States.
5. 23 of the 30 billion animals living on U.S. farms are chickens.
6. More than half of all entrees ordered in U.S. fast food chains, hotels, motels, and restaurants are some version of fried chicken.
7. In addition to chicken being the favorite food of many, chicken soup is a time-honored folk remedy often served up to treat colds.
8. An entire line of best-selling books, "Chicken Soup for the Soul," sprang from the popularity of this soothing broth.

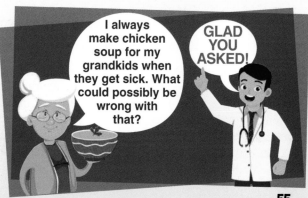

What's Unhealthy About Chicken Farms?

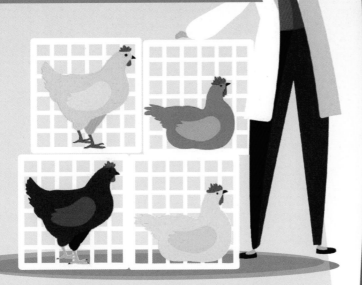

MANY FACTORY FARM ANIMALS, INCLUDING CHICKENS, ARE FORCED TO GROW UP TO 3 TIMES FASTER THAN NATURE INTENDED

Size of Broiler Chickens Bred in the Following Years:

1957 0.9 kg

1978 1.8 kg

2005 4.2 kg

- On factory farms, chickens are selectively bred and fed for abnormally fast growth, leading to a number of health challenges.
- Literally millions of chickens are penned in small spaces inside large buildings without sunlight, fresh air, or freedom to move.
- Chickens on these farms are in a continual state of stress, which is very immunosuppressive.
- Poor sanitation and waste management on factory farms leads to contamination of rivers and sometimes vegetables by bacteria such as *Campylobacter, E. coli, Listeria,* and *Salmonella*.

Chicken Farms and Bird Flu in the News

"A highly contagious and deadly form of avian influenza is spreading rapidly in Europe, putting the poultry industry on alert with previous outbreaks in mind that saw tens of millions of birds culled and significant economic losses. The disease, commonly called bird flu, has been found in France, the Netherlands, Germany, Britain, Belgium, Denmark, Ireland, Sweden and, for the first time this week in Croatia, Slovenia and Poland, after severely hitting Russia, Kazakhstan and Israel. The vast majority of cases are in migrating wild birds but outbreaks have been reported on farms, leading to the death or culling of at least 1.6 million chickens and ducks so far around the region." — Reuters, November 26, 2020

AND THE WINNER IS...
Chicken Tops the Wrong List

- According to the CDC, chicken causes 12% of foodborne illnesses.

- Each year, 76 million Americans become ill and 5,000 die from food borne illness.

Japan's Bird Flu Outbreak Worsens with Record Cullings

"A bird flu outbreak in Japan worsened on Thursday with farms in two more prefectures slaughtering chicken in a record cull of poultry as the government ordered the disinfection of all chicken farms. Highly pathogenic bird flu, a H5 subtype most likely brought by migrating birds from the Asian/European continent, has spread to eight of Japan's 47 prefectures. While officials say it is not possible for people to catch avian influenza from eggs or meat of infected chickens, they are concerned about the virus making a "species jump" to humans and causing a pandemic like the novel coronavirus." — Reuters, December 9, 2020

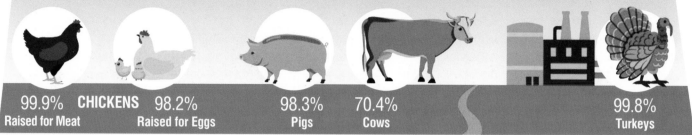

Unfortunately, factory farming — and the pandemic potential it brings — isn't limited to chickens. In the United States, the vast majority of farmed animals live on factory farms.

99.9% **CHICKENS** Raised for Meat — 98.2% Raised for Eggs — 98.3% **Pigs** — 70.4% **Cows** — 99.8% **Turkeys**

Viruses that Leaped from Pigs to Humans

NIPAH VIRUS: First identified in 1998, the Nipah Virus is an emerging disease that causes severe illness in both pigs and humans. The virus may be contracted by touching infected bats or pigs, eating fruit contaminated by infected bats, or contact with infected persons. The death rate for Nipah Virus is 40-70%.

SWINE FLU (H1N1 VIRUS): The first outbreak of this virus, which originated on a crowded pig farm in Mexico, occurred in 2009. Estimates of worldwide deaths range from 151,000 to 575,000.

Viruses that Could Leap from Pigs to Humans, but Haven't Yet Made the Jump

SWINE ACUTE DIARRHEA SYNDROME (SADS): First discovered in 2017, SADS is a coronavirus that results in death for up to 90% of piglets who contract it. Based on in vitro testing, scientists believe that humans are susceptible to this deadly virus.

PORCINE EPIDEMIC DIARRHEA SYNDROME (PED VIRUS): First identified in 2014, PED killed more than a million piglets in the United States that year. Also a coronavirus, this deadly disease has a mortality rate of up to 100% for piglets under 7 days old.

The Straight "Skinny" on Factory Pig Farms

- Many pigs on factory farms live out their lives in pens that are only 18-24 inches wide, or metal "gestation" crates.
- In these crates, the pigs cannot walk or turn around. There is barely enough room for them to stand or sit down.
- These overcrowded, underventilated conditions are very stressful (and therefore immune suppressing) for the pigs.
- Many pigs living on factory farms contract leg and bone problems from being forced to lay on concrete.
- More than 80% of pigs have pneumonia at the time they are slaughtered.
- Cramming large numbers of pigs together creates the "perfect" conditions for diseases to be transmitted or mutate into more dangerous strains.

6 Reasons to "Steer" Clear of Dairy

While cows aren't as closely linked to potential viruses as some other farm animals, there are plenty of health-related reasons for concern. Following is an overview:

1. Despite modern sanitation efforts, outbreaks of illness due to dairy-related foodborne pathogens still occur. *Listeria, E. coli,* and *Salmonella* are some of the more common foodborne outbreaks associated with dairy.

2. Due to their elevated fat content, dairy products often contain high concentrations of pesticides.

3. Because of the significant antibiotic doses given to dairy cattle to keep them "healthier" on crowded factory farms, dairy products include low level doses of antibiotics which may lead to allergic reactions, antibiotic resistance, or other side effects.

4. Dairy products (even organic ones) contain significant amounts of hormones such as estrogen and progesterone. Milk consumption has been linked to increased levels of estradiol and progesterone in the blood, decreased testosterone levels in men, early sexual maturation in children, and other hormone-related disorders.

5. Casein from dairy increases the risk of cancer, diabetes, Multiple Sclerosis, and allergies.

6. Consuming dairy products is bad for bone health. The U.S., which has one of the highest levels of dairy consumption in the world, also has one of the highest rates of hip fractures.

ANTIBIOTICS AND FACTORY FARMS: What You Should Know

- Antibiotics are medicines used to treat infections caused by bacteria. Antibiotics kill the bacteria (not the viruses).
- Antibiotic resistance arises when bacteria change to protect themselves against an antibiotic.
- Factory farm animals, which often fall sick due to stress and overcrowding, are fed antibiotics to make them grow faster and keep them in a basic state of "wellness" whether they are sick or not.
- While antibiotics do wipe out some intestinal invaders, they also deplete good intestinal bacteria and damage the immune system.
- Each use of antibiotics makes them less effective the next time around. As a result, more and stronger drugs are always needed.

ANTIBIOTIC RESISTANCE: How it Happens

STEP 1: Farm animals are fed antibiotics freely regardless of need.

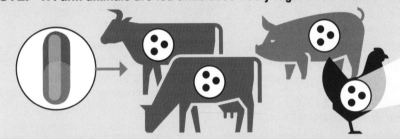

STEP 2: Mutated forms of the bacteria become antibiotic resistant.

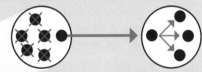

The antibiotics protect the farm animals from known strains of bacteria.

Mutated forms of bacteria resist the antibiotic and infect the animals.

STEP 3: The resistant bacteria is spread to humans through…

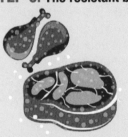

Meat and other animal products

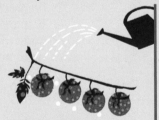

Produce that has been contaminated through water or soil

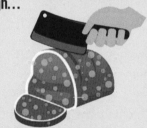

Prepared food that has been contaminated by unsanitary surfaces

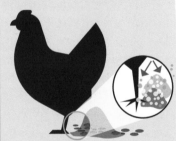

The environment (when infected by animal excrement)

STEP 4: Humans who get sick from the resistant bacteria are treated with the same antibiotic the pathogen has learned to resist.

STEP 5: The antibiotic is ineffective against that pathogen, since it has already developed immunity.

 ## Action Plan

→ Consider your current diet. If you are eating forms of meat that may increase your risk of disease, look for and try out some "eat this not that" alternatives that might appeal to you.

→ If you think curtailing chicken, dairy, or other animal product consumption would be too hard, watch some documentaries on factory farming. For anyone who loves animals, these can be highly motivational in terms of positive change.

→ If you are consuming foods that might include antibiotics, consider what alternatives you might try.

PURGE YOUR PALATE
Of Pangolins, Primates, and Penguins

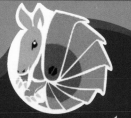

Although bushmeat most often refers to African animals killed for food, it is also a catchall phrase for the meat of any wild or exotic animals.

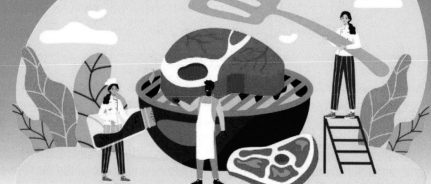

5 Facts You Should Know About Bushmeat and Other Exotic Cuisine

1 "Bushmeat" is a major food source in the undeveloped world.

Bushmeat is the primary source of animal protein, plus a valuable, cash-earning commodity, for many of the world's poor living in the humid tropical forest regions of Africa, Latin America and Asia.

2 Bushmeat has been closely linked to Emerging Infectious Diseases.

Hunting and eating bushmeat has been linked to the origin of deadly new diseases such as Ebola, AIDS, and SARS.

3 One person eating a monkey can put the world at risk.

You don't have to eat or even come anywhere near bushmeat to catch a virus from it. You just have to come near a person who did. Which, in this age of globalization, isn't hard.

4 The world is one mutation away from disaster.

Because many viruses have such a high mutation rate, they can rapidly evolve to yield new, unforeseen (and potentially lethal) variants. The AIDS virus, which is believed to have gotten its start when someone ate a chimpanzee, was rapidly spread by other methods once it made the "jump" to humans.

5 The best strategy is not only to keep the "exotics" from your plate, but also to build your immune system.

We can't control what others eat. In this globalized world, we can't even control who we might "rub shoulders" with. But we can make socially responsible choices about what to put on our own plates. We can also put our bodies in the very best shape possible to ward off any disease.

CHAPTER 15

So Why Do People Hunt — And Eat — Bush Meat?

If you don't have a taste for tarantulas, you might wonder "why in the world" people would eat such a thing. Following are the reasons why, despite legislation from various countries, many people (and cultures) persist in hunting and consuming exotic meat — even if they have to go underground:

- Bushmeat is a major protein source for many of the poorest and hungriest nations of the world.
- In countries where bushmeat is viewed as a delicacy, being able to afford it is linked to wealth and prestige.
- Hunting bushmeat is a source of entertainment or game for some tourists.

What People are Eating — And How That Has Led to Disease

Its hard to quantify the amount of bushmeat being taken, because the numbers are so immense. Worldwide, its estimated that more than 1,000 animal species are being hunted for bushmeat. Researchers tracking what was served at a set of nine restaurants specializing in exotic meats documented that those restaurants alone, over a 6-month period, served up 376 different types of mammals, plus 8 reptile species, on their menu. Much of the meat being served comes from rare and endangered species. Following is an overview of some of the most popular, with an eye to those that have also been closely linked to disease:

Monkeys and their Cousins
(including Baboons, Chimpanzees, Gorillas, and More)

- The meat of monkeys and others primates is one of the most common and popular forms of bushmeat.
- Similarities between the biology of primates and humans makes it easier for bacteria (and zoonotic diseases) to jump from monkeys to humans, and vice versa.
- The deadly AIDS virus, which has taken the lives of more than 32 million people worldwide, has been traced to human contact (either eating or another form of contamination) with a chimpanzee.
- The origin of the Ebola virus, which most often affects humans and non-human primates (chimpanzees, gorillas, and monkeys), has also been traced to human consumption or contact with a primate.

Armadillos

- A high percentage of armadillos are carriers of leprosy, a chronic disease that leads to disfigurement and nerve damage. Although percentages vary by region, 62% of armadillos in the western Pará state of Brazil were found to be infected with the disease.
- Researchers have reported that human contact with wild armadillos — including eating the meat — has led to human cases of leprosy in Brazil.
- Only about 200 cases of leprosy are diagnosed in the United States each year. To put this into perspective, in Brazil, where leprosy-infected armadillos are handled, hunted, and eaten, clinicians diagnose about 25,000 cases of leprosy each year.

Civets

- The civet cat (which actually is more like a mongoose than a cat) is a popular commodity in Chinese animal markets.
- In addition to being raised for meat, civets produce the most expensive coffee in the world.
- "Fox dung coffee," as their culinary specialty is called, is produced by feeding coffee beans to captive civets, then recovering the partially digested beans from their feces.
- The SARs epidemic, which infected more than 8,000 people worldwide and took the lives of close to 800, was traced by researchers to this animal.

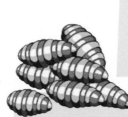

Maggots

In some cultures, maggots are considered to be a delicacy or even a superfood. This is problematic because:

- Maggots are often infected by flies, which bring them harmful bacteria (such as *Salmonella* and *E. coli*).
- Humans who eat maggots can get infected with "Intestinal Myiasis," in which case fly larvae infest their bodies, feeding on tissue both inside and out.
- Ingestion of maggots can also result in food poisoning.

Alligators

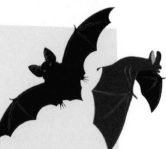

- Because their environment is less controlled than domestic farm animals, alligators are susceptible to parasites, viruses, prions, and other hazards not as readily found in farmed meats.
- Researchers have found that alligators can amplify West Nile virus, serve as a reservoir host, and pass the infection to humans. (West Nile Virus is currently the leading cause of mosquito-borne disease in the United States.)

Pangolins

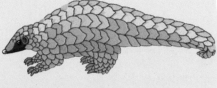

- Pangolins, scaly anteaters that look like a cross between a pine cone and a sloth, are known for rolling up in a ball when they sense a threat.
- Pangolin meat is prized as a delicacy and as a component in traditional Chinese medicine.
- The high demand for both the meat and scales of these creatures has made them the most trafficked mammal in the world.
- Researchers believe that pangolins were at least partially responsible for the start of COVID-19.

Fruit Bats

- Fruit bats are a popular menu item in parts of China, Thailand, Guam and even Australia, where they might be stir fried, dropped into boiling milk, roasted, put into soups, or cooked any number of other ways.
- As a natural reservoir for viruses, fruit bats (also known as flying foxes) have been involved in at least three emerging zoonotic diseases in recent years.
- Consumption of fruit bats on the island of Guam is blamed for causing a sudden appearance of a Parkinson's disease-like syndrome in the 1970's.
- Researchers have traced strains of SARS, Ebola and other emerging diseases to fruit bats.

The animals listed are just a few of the hundreds of types of creatures being farmed, hunted, and eaten on a regular basis. While these practices are problematic enough, even more trouble begins when many species of wild animals are brought together into "wet" or "live animal" markets.

What is wrong with wet markets?

- Wild animals that appear healthy often harbor diseases that can make other animals — and humans — sick.
- Wildlife that would not ordinarily be in close contact (e.g. pangolins, civets, and bats) are kept in confined spaces, often in poor health, with little access to water or food.
- When these animals are slaughtered, viruses continue to mutate in their dead flesh. This is one way in which viruses evolve, spread, and eventually try to make the "leap" to a human host.
- Because of these and other factors, live animal markets are a major source of new viruses, including ones that cause zoonotic diseases.

What is a wet market?

- Similar to a farmer's market, a wet market is a large collection of open-air stalls where individual vendors sell fresh seafood, meat, fruits, and vegetables.
- Some cultures prefer to shop 2-3 times per week for fruits, vegetables, and freshly slaughtered meat. To serve this market, hundreds of live animals are kept, and slaughtered, on site.
- Such markets acquired the name "wet" because fish sellers regularly hosed down the floors of their areas.

Some cultures have factory farms. Some cultures have wet markets. In the end, the net result is the same. Too many animals, too close together, in a stressful "cauldron of contagion" ideally suited to foment new strains of disease.

5 Ways Humans Get Diseases From Animals

1. By direct contact with the saliva, urine, or feces of infected animals.

2. By being in areas where infected animals live, or touching something contaminated by an infected animal.

3. By being bitten or scratched by an infected animal.

4. By eating contaminated animal products, or animals products that have been improperly handled or cooked.

5. Through a "vector" such as a fly or a mosquito.

Common Diseases Passed from Animals to Humans

ANTHRAX: A bacterial infection which affects domestic and wild animals, anthrax infects humans when they:
- Breathe anthrax spores
- Eat food or drink water contaminated with anthrax spores
- Get a skin cut or scrape which is then infected by anthrax spores

AVIAN INFLUENZA: A viral infection that affects birds, then humans and animals, Avian Influenza was first discovered among poultry handlers in Hong Kong in 1997.

EBOLA VIRUS: Believed to have originated from African fruit bats, this virus infects wild animals first, and then is transmitted to humans. After the first human is infected, it spreads from human to human.

RABIES: This viral disease is usually transmitted to humans through the bites or scratches of infected animals, such as cats, dogs, raccoons, and skunks.

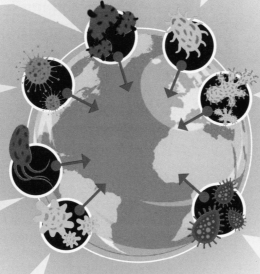

HIV (AIDS): AIDS is the late stage of HIV infection that occurs when the body's immune system is badly damaged due to the HIV virus. Although spread most commonly through human body fluids, the original HIV virus is believed to have been transmitted through human contact with a chimpanzee.

SEVERE ACUTE RESPIRATORY SYNDROME (SARS): First identified as a virus in 2003, SARS is thought to have originated with bats.

MIDDLE EAST RESPIRATORY SYNDROME (MERS): First reported in Saudi Arabia in 2012, MERS is a severe respiratory illness thought to have originated with camels.

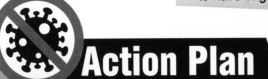

Action Plan

If you have a taste for "wild," unusual or exotic meat, or are:

→ Using traditional remedies that contain unusual ingredients drawn from some animal part, or

→ Handling or otherwise coming in contact with these types of meats in your line of work,

→ Consider how you can reduce your risk of contracting a zoonotic disease through contact with animals, then make and implement a plan.

INFECTION PROTECTION

Lifesaving Things You Should Know

How Your Immune System Functions — And Why You Should Care

YOUR IMMUNE SYSTEM IS:

- Working constantly to protect your body against infection, injury, and disease.
- Your body's built-in defense system, equipped with the power not only to protect, but to heal.

When functioning properly, your immune system will identify and attack a variety of threats, including bacteria, parasites, and viruses, all while telling the difference between these threats and your body's own tissue.

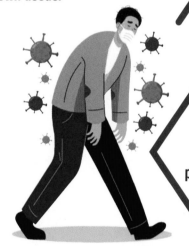

When things go haywire, your immune system either doesn't recognize a threat right away, or isn't prepared to fight it. Worse yet, it might even attack your own organs.

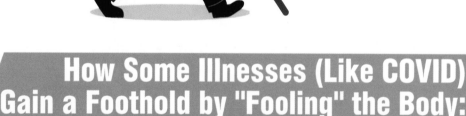

How Some Illnesses (Like COVID) Gain a Foothold by "Fooling" the Body:

- When your immune system is functioning normally, your body will respond to "invaders" by releasing chemicals called interferons.
- As a first line of defense, interferons signal to the immune system and the rest of the body that an attack is now underway.
- Unfortunately, COVID-19 has an amazing capacity to switch off this natural warning system.
- With the warning system switched off, the interferons fail to "interfere" and the immune system is lulled into complacency.
- Because the infected person feels basically fine, they continue their normal routine. Meanwhile, the "silent" infection grows stronger and stronger.
- By the time the immune system recognizes that it is under attack, it's got a blood battle on its hands. Literally.

NOTE: COVID-19 isn't the only disease that tampers with the "signal calling" interferons. The MERS, SARS, and HIV viruses, in addition to the disease of Multiple Sclerosis, also shut down interferons as they move in to attack.

CHAPTER 16

QUESTION: Why do some people's immune systems rise up and fight off a virus, when others do not?

ANSWER: Because they have plenty of interferons in their bodies at the start of the infection.

When a Virus STRIKES:

 Interferons in the infected cell are activated and released.

 Interferons sound the alarm, calling backup cells to the area of the infection.

 Immune cells respond to the call by helping to heal infected cells and protecting cells that haven't yet been infected.

 Together, the cells stop the virus from spreading.

Why Interferons are So Important

- When the immune system is strong and interferon levels are high at the beginning, the infection is recognized, a healthy response kicks in, and the infection is defeated.
- The people who have trouble are the ones whose white blood cells aren't secreting enough interferon when the infection arrives.
- With a lack of "signal callers" to "interfere" with the infection by alerting the rest of the body, the immune system is in a diminished, vulnerable state.
- By the time the immune system "catches on" and sends out a "Mayday" signal, the virus has already gained a very strong foothold in the body.
- The harmful "Cytokine Storm" which overwhelms the system wouldn't have happened if the immune system was primed with interferons in the beginning. The interferons really are key.

Understanding Cytokine Storms

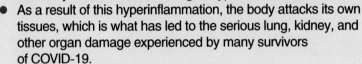

- When the body's immune system goes into overdrive to fight an infection, that response is known as a "cytokine storm."
- During a cytokine storm, uncontrolled levels of cytokines activate too many immune cells, leading to hyperinflammation.
- As a result of this hyperinflammation, the body attacks its own tissues, which is what has led to the serious lung, kidney, and other organ damage experienced by many survivors of COVID-19.

NOTE: Though they have received much publicity due to COVID-19, cytokine storms have also been documented in cases of influenza, SARS, and MERS.

Interferon Lessons from Bats

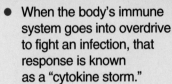

- Bats can carry many viruses in their bodies which are extremely dangerous to humans without being harmed themselves.
- A huge factor behind the immunity of bats to the deadly diseases they carry is the large amount of interferons they produce.
- Some researchers believe that, if human beings have more interferons early on, they (like bats) would be much better equipped to fend off COVID-19 as well as other ailments.

Inflammation's Role in a Cytokine Storm

- Whenever the body is fighting an infection, inflammation is the normal response.
- In its efforts to fight off the invader, the body sends extra blood flow to the site of the infection.
- Extra antibodies and proteins are also released.
- When the immune system is impaired (e.g. interferons aren't primed and ready), the body issues a delayed inflammatory response.
- Though delayed, the inflammatory response quickly ramps up.
- This inflammatory flood, the "cytokine storm," destroys tissue but not the infection.

Infection Protection

 QUESTION: If I have a stronger immune system, doesn't that mean I will have a stronger cytokine storm?

ANSWER: No. A stronger and healthier immune system will recognize and fight the infection earlier, which will prevent the body from "falling behind" and overcompensating with a damaging cytokine storm.

PEOPLE WITH THE MOST SERIOUS HEALTH PROBLEMS HAVE BEEN THE ONES MOST LIKELY TO DEVELOP SEVERE CASES OF COVID-19. BECAUSE THEIR IMMUNE SYSTEMS ARE ALREADY COMPROMISED BY INFLAMMATION, THEY ARE LESS ABLE TO FEND OFF NEW THREATS.

In one study, researchers from the American Institute of Lifestyle Medicine documented that 86.2% of 5,489 hospitalized COVID-19 patients had at least one comorbidity.

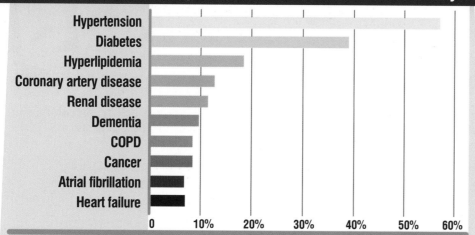

 QUESTION: What does this mean to me?

ANSWER: Many lifestyle diseases can be reversed or significantly improved through healthier choices. This book is a call to each of us to do all that we can to bolster our immune systems. In that way, we can better prepare our bodies to fend off any threats or invaders.

In 99 different countries, many of the patients hospitalized with COVID-19 had underlying health conditions.

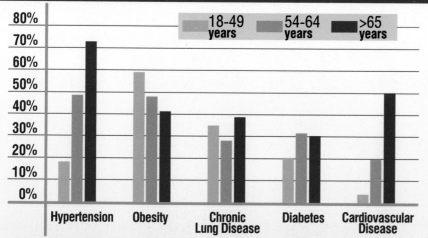

NOTE: Based on data from the COVID-19-Associated Hospitalization Surveillance Network for patients hospitalized in 99 countries in 14 states from March 1-13, 2020. SOURCE: MMWR. 2020 Apr 8:69(early release):1-7

A Vaccine is Not a Magic Bullet...

- Some people see a vaccine as a license to continue unhealthy lifestyle practices without fear of COVID-19 or similar threats.
- This is a terrible mistake, since poor choices can undo whatever good a vaccine may have done.
- A recent study, where COVID-19 vaccinated persons who didn't sleep well produced fewer antibodies than sound sleepers, illustrates this point.
- It remains up to all of us to make the best choices so we can enhance our health.

QUESTION: Why has so much emphasis been put on masks, social distancing, and vaccines— while not much has been said about the immune-boosting strategies emphasized in this book?

 ANSWER: Making lifestyle changes requires both effort and commitment. Many people wish they could just "take a pill" or "get a shot" and COVID-19, or similar threats, would simply go away.

Immune-boosting Lifestyle Strategies

QUESTION: What about supplements?

ANSWER: Evidence-based research does support the use of some supplements against COVID-19. Following is a list to consider:

MELATONIN: Well-known for its sleep-promoting properties, melatonin is also a natural antiviral, anti-inflammatory, and antioxidant. Research suggests that melatonin supplements, especially for older adults, may be protective against viruses and pathogens.

N-ACETYL CYSTEINE (NAC): A derivative of the L-cysteine (an amino acid), NAC helps to boost glutathione levels, which are important for their immune system support. NAC is especially helpful to the lungs, where it reduces inflammation and inhibits the replication of viruses.

SELENIUM: Researchers believe that selenium, a trace mineral, may help protect the immune system against harmful virus mutations. You can get the Recommended Daily Allowance (RDA) of this important mineral by eating 1-2 Brazil nuts daily. Whole grains and seeds are also good sources of selenium.

VITAMIN D: This important vitamin, which is really a hormone, helps reduce the risk of a cytokine storm by regulating immune system response. Research has shown that the vast majority of COVID-19 fatalities were low on vitamin D.

ZINC: Another trace mineral, zinc helps the immune system to protect against invading viruses and bacteria.

 ## Action Plan

→ Think about the health of your own immune system. Is it functioning as well as you think it could? If not, what could you do to help it work better?

→ Do you have, personally, any underlying conditions or comorbidities that make you more vulnerable to viruses and/or pathogens that might come along? If there are lifestyle choices you can make that would improve your situation, make a plan to get started.

→ If you have been vaccinated and feel the vaccine is a cure-all, consider re-thinking that position and recommitting to doing all you can to make the vaccine more effective.

→ Do some research on the supplements suggested above, to see if any might be helpful in your particular situation.

GET OUT OF YOUR HEAD
The Magic of Self-Control

Self-control is one of the most important qualities needed to live a healthy, happy life. It is also a key factor to success in making the lifestyle changes needed to boost the immune system. That means there are life-or-death implications involved. Yet most people don't like the terms self-control, self-discipline, or anything remotely related. To counter the negativity associated with the very idea of self-control, psychologists have even coined a new term: self-regulation.

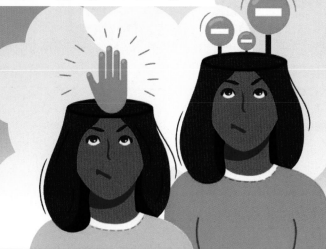

What does all this mean to you, in the setting of boosting your immune system? Here's what you need to know:

Self-control: Regulating what one feels and does, being disciplined, and controlling one's appetites and emotions.

Self-regulation: The consistent and appropriate application of self-control.

People who have good self-discipline are better able to:

- Control emotions, desires, impulses, and behavior.
- Resist short-term temptations in favor of prioritizing actions that will help to achieve longer-term goals.
- Make better decisions.
- Handle pressure that he or she might encounter.
- Deal with diverse and/ or challenging personalities, no matter how difficult they may be.

NOTE:

While some psychologists view the term "self-control" as outdated and judgmental, it doesn't have to be. In order to have the happiest life — as well as boost your immune system by taking some of the lifestyle "polar plunges" in this book, you'll need to make some choices. And self-control, regardless of whether you call it grit, perseverance, self-discipline, temperance, or some other term, will need to be part of the equation.

So how do I get self-control?

Read on, Honey…

In this book, we've focused on helping you build a stronger immune system. As part of that challenge, we've suggested plenty of "Action Steps" that you can take. It all might seem a bit overwhelming, especially if you need a "cosmic shift" in your life. To make things easier we've divided our self-control building plan into the familiar sections often used to advertise an event:

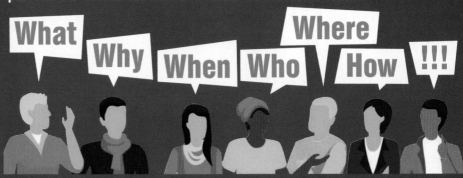

What **Why** **When** **Who** **Where** **How** **!!!**

We have mixed them around a little, to make them work more smoothly for this process. So if you'd like to have more self-discipline but feel you're running on "empty," here's how to get started!

Small Actions
x
Consistency
=
BIG CHANGE

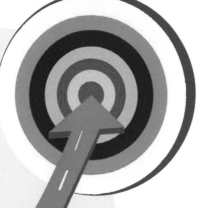

With self-discipline, almost anything is possible.
— Theodore Roosevelt

SUCC ESS

Making positive changes can take a lot of self-discipline. Fortunately, while it can be hard to muster up the willpower to take action, there are many things you can to do make things much easier. This chapter includes a list of seven strategies to consider.

Step One
Know Your "What"

To begin, we recommend that you choose just one thing. Trying to make a lot of changes "cold turkey" doesn't work well for most people. Conquering just one thing will actually build your willpower muscle, making you more able to go on to the next. While we wouldn't discourage anyone who feels a need to go "all out" with lifestyle changes, for purposes of this plan we encourage you to:

1. Choose one thing (e.g. lifestyle factor that will boost your immune system) that you would really like to change.

2. Make that one thing something that you feel is not only doable but will be very impactful for your life.

3. As you get started and build up your self-regulatory momentum, focus on that one thing every day.

Step Two
Know Your "Why"

A desire to have a stronger immune system is just one of many reasons why you might want to make multiple changes in your life. Other reasons that resonate with many include:

- Living the highest quality of life, actively and fulfilled, for as long as possible.
- Being there for parents, a spouse, children, grandchildren, or others you love.
- Taking care of yourself and retaining independence as long as you can.
- Just flat-out feeling better!
- Having a strong reason to wake up in the morning (known as the Ikigai in Japan).

Whatever your "why's" might be, you will be much more likely to stick to your plan if they are clearly in view. That is why we recommend, as part of this step, that you write down the reasons behind your new goals. For this exercise, it can also be helpful to visualize how you will benefit by this change. Studies have shown that willpower lasts longer for people who are motivated by a vision of the positive results they hope to obtain.

Success follows when
YOU DEFINE WHAT
inspires YOU
MOTIVATES YOU
AND FIRES YOU UP!
What's your why?

When you know why you do what you do even the toughest days become easier!

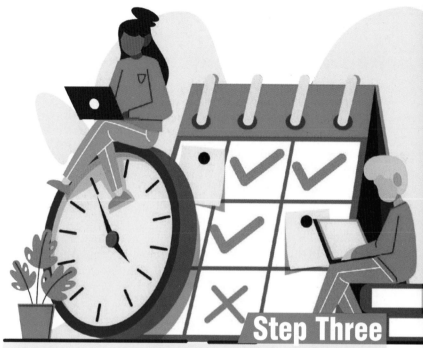

Step Three
Know Your "When"

People who set goals and actually achieve them put those goals on their calendar. There is just something about setting a start date that makes it more real. Also, researchers have found that people who set a start date for any new regimen are more likely to follow through on their goals. So go ahead. Now's the time to put that goal on the calendar!

Step Four Know Your "Who"

At first glance, this one might seem easy. Your "who" will be you, of course! There's a bit more to it than that, however. An old adage says: "if you want to go fast, go by yourself – but if you want to go far, go together." Researchers have found that those with social support are more likely to stick to and accomplish their goals. Here are some ways to get that support:

1. Surround yourself with self-disciplined people. The influence of friends who are already achieving what you are trying to do can have a powerful positive impact.

2. If you have family and friends who will be supportive, tell them about your goals and ask for encouragement. If your closest associates are continually dragging you down, that will be a problem. We don't recommend "trading in" family, but you could "trade in" a few friends. Or make some new ones, at least.

What if you live in the country, with no stellar, positive or healthy friend prospects in sight? Here's where good books and videos come in. You can associate with the most successful people on this planet, people who have conquered whatever it is you are fighting, in the comfort of your own home. Even if you don't know them personally, you can watch their videos, read their books, and be inspired.

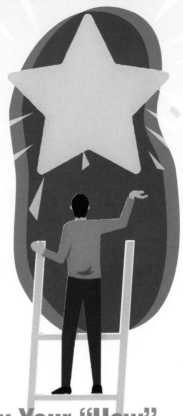

CHAPTER 17

Step Five
Know Your "Where"

This section might better be entitled, "Know Your Where Nots." If you are trying to quit drinking but drive by the town bar every night on the way home from work, its time for a different route. If you walk by the office snack bar every time you go to the restroom, look for the long way around. For this step, take some time and think of "where" you are most likely to struggle with whatever habit you wish to form or break. Then make a plan. By avoiding some places entirely, you can enhance your probability of success by reducing the drain — and strain — on your willpower muscle.

Step Six   Know Your "How"

We've already talked about the "Why," "Who," "When," and "Where." The "How" adds more practical actions to the steps you have already taken above. Here are some "How's" to consider when making your plan:

PLAN AHEAD FOR TEMPTATION. This means to foresee situations that might break your resolve and have a plan for how to deal with them. For example, if someone offers you a soda, you might plan to ask for sparkling water or plain water instead.

REMOVE THE TEMPTATIONS FROM YOUR OFFICE OR HOME. If you simply hide your "downfalls," you will still know where they are and be tempted in your weak moments. So get rid of them entirely, if you can.

LEARN HOW TO "PAIR" ACTIVITIES. Many people have been able to motivate themselves to do things they didn't want to do (e.g. taking a walk) with something they like (e.g. visiting with a friend).

SPREAD VISUAL CUES AROUND YOUR OFFICE OR HOME. Meaningful cues posted around an office or home can be a great boost to willpower.

BUILD REWARDS INTO YOUR PLAN. Think of some healthy treats and breaks to reward yourself when you reach certain milestones or goals.

Step Seven
Put Your Plan into Action

As your well-thought-out plan swings into action, consider adding the following steps to bolster your odds of success:

EAT HEALTHY AND SLEEP WELL. Both diet and sleeping habits will impact your ability to exercise self-control.

KEEP FOCUSED ON YOUR "WHY'S." You'll need those motivational reasons for sticking with your plan until it becomes natural to you.

KEEP YOUR BLOOD SUGAR STABLE. Studies have shown that willpower "fails" are often tied to low blood glucose levels. If you sense a blood sugar dip coming on and don't want to snack, one trick used by some is to drink hot water with lemon juice and a tablespoon of honey stirred in.

AVOID ALCOHOL CONSUMPTION. Research shows alcohol can compromise self-discipline by reducing the ability to reflect on the consequences of potential actions.

BE NICE TO YOURSELF. Don't fret if you make a mistake. Forgive yourself quickly and move on with a new beginning.

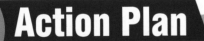

Action Plan

→ Scan the chapters you have read thus far in this book. Are there some things you would like to change? If so, is there one thing you feel you could focus on to start?

→ Follow the seven steps in this chapter to form a plan and implement it for the area you wish to improve first.

BRUSH YOUR TEETH:
The Dental — Immune System Link

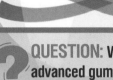

Startling Stats about Gum Health and Severe COVID-19

In a recent study, researchers found that people with advanced gum disease who contracted COVID-19 were:

- 4 times more likely to be transferred into Intensive Care
- 5 times more likely to be put on a ventilator
- 9 times more likely to die

The same patients also had significantly higher levels of C-Reactive Protein (a marker for inflammation) than patients whose COVID-19 illnesses were not as severe.

 QUESTION: Why do people with advanced gum disease get the most severe cases of COVID-19?

ANSWER: Because oral (mouth) health is closely connected to the health of the entire body. When there is inflammation in the gums, you can be sure that there is inflammation in the gut and also other areas of the body.

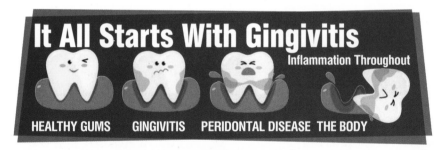

It All Starts With Gingivitis — Inflammation Throughout

HEALTHY GUMS   GINGIVITIS   PERIDONTAL DISEASE   THE BODY

Other Disease-related Dental Facts

- Gum disease is one of the most common chronic diseases in the world. It's been estimated that 20-50% of the world population suffers from gum disease. Some studies in the United States and Great Britain have suggested that 50-90% of the adult population suffers from some level of gingivitus.
- When the body is fighting infections in multiple areas, fewer disease-attacking white blood cells are available in the mouth. This leaves fewer resources to eradicate incoming threats.
- The journal Oral Disease reported that, due to the high incidence of tongue ulcers, mouth rash, and lip necrosis associated with COVID-19, the mouth is considered to be a main source of coronavirus infection and transmission.
- The widespread practice of mask-wearing for extended periods of time has brought on a new malady, known as "Mask Mouth," with an accompanying set of dental challenges (see the following page).

GUM DISEASE AND RESPIRATORY ILLNESS: HOW THINGS GET STARTED

Bad bacteria, viruses, or pathogens that cause respiratory infections get inside the body when people inhale fine droplets from the mouth and throat into the lungs. After traveling down to the lungs, these unhealthy invaders breed and multiply. As the body rushes "fighter cells" to the area, inflammation sets in. Eventually, if the flames aren't calmed down, tissue is damaged. As the American Academy of Periodontology has reported, "Bacteria that grow in the oral cavity can be aspirated into the lung to cause respiratory diseases such as pneumonia, especially in people with periodontal disease." It should be no surprise, then, that multiple scientific studies have found a very strong association between poor oral health and bacterial "super infections."

The "Mask Mouth" Conundrum

Wearing a mask, especially in confined spaces where germs may abound, can definitely impact the transmission of airborne bacteria, viruses, and pathogens. The N95 mask in particular, which is worn by surgeons worldwide, gets its name from the fact that it filters out 95% of airborne particles. While wearing masks for short periods of time is harmless enough, wearing masks for extended periods of time can be problematic for the following reasons:

- **Shallower mouth breathing:** Mask wearing tends to encourage mouth breathing. This decreases the amount of saliva and leads to "dry mouth," which creates a perfect breeding ground for viruses and bacteria to grow, thereby increasing the risk of bad breath, tooth decay, and infections.
- **Dehydration:** Wearing a mask leads some to drink less water than usual, which once again leads to dry mouth.
- **Recycled air:** Wearing a mask results in more carbon dioxide than usual being trapped in the mouth. These slightly elevated carbon dioxide levels increase the acidity of the mouth's microbiome, raising the risk of gum disease and other inflammatory conditions.

The "conundrum" is that, by negatively impacting the type and amount of bacteria in your mouth, mask wearing can trigger a chain of events that weakens the immune system, lowering resistance to the very disease the mask was intended to prevent. By some estimates, 50% of patients being seen by dentists today are suffering from some degree of "mask mouth."

> *Every time you swallow, you are seeding your gastrointestinal tract with bacteria, fungi, and viruses from your mouth — 140 billion per day, to be exact.*
> — Cass Nelson-Dooley, Heal Your Oral Microbiome

The Mouth-Gut Connection: A Major Player in Overall Health

While most people understand the rather direct connection between the mouth and the gut, not as many understand the huge impact that the bacteria residing in the mouth have on the gut, the immune system, and overall health. For example:

- Just like your gut, your mouth is a "bacterial playground" with literally hundreds of types of bacteria living inside.
- When a virus meets up with the bacteria in your mouth, it can feed on that bacteria to grow and multiply.
- Bad bacteria love junk food, which is why the extra comfort food many people are eating to soothe them through the stress of the pandemic is doubly harmful.
- When a virus enters your mouth, it doesn't just "stay put." Rather, it travels throughout your entire body, compromising your immune system.
- If your gums become inflamed with bacteria, your whole body can also become inflamed. This is the reason why diseases of inflammation have been so closely linked to gum (periodontal) disease.

4 Ways to Reduce Mask Mouth

1. PRACTICE GOOD ORAL HYGIENE:

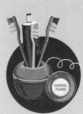

It's a good practice to brush and floss twice daily. To keep your mouth clear of left-behind food particles, it's also a good idea to rinse your mouth out whenever you finish eating.

2. TREAT GUM DISEASE:

If you suspect gum disease, visit your dentist and start treatment right away.

3. WATCH YOUR DIET:

Some foods, such as alcohol, junk food, and sugar, feed bad bacteria. Cutting down on such foods and eating healthier will give your good bacteria a boost.

4. KEEP MASKS FRESH AND CLEAN:

If you don't wash or replace masks, bacteria from your breath can grow on the mask and wait there for you to breathe them back in again!

45%
OF THE BACTERIA IN THE MOUTH ARE ALSO FOUND IN THE GUT.

80%
OF AMERICANS SUFFER FROM SOME FORM OF GUM DISEASE.

Health Challenges Linked to Gum Disease and an Unhealthy Gut Microbiome

Researchers have reported that when dental health is lacking, there is less health-promoting nitric oxide in the blood. Health challenges that researchers have linked to gum disease include:

- Inflammatory Bowel Disease
- Kidney Disease
- Liver Cancer
- Obesity
- Osteoporosis
- Poor Immune System Function
- Pre-term Births
- Respiratory Diseases

- Alzheimer's Disease
- Arthritis
- Anxiety
- Cirrhosis of the Liver
- Colon Cancer
- Depression
- Diabetes
- Gut Cancer
- Heart Disease
- Hypertension

STUDIES SHOW THAT MEN WITH GUM DISEASE ARE:

30% more likely to get blood cancers
59% more likely to get kidney cancer
54% more likely to get pancreatic cancer

Gum Disease Symptoms

Because gum disease is often silent, many people don't realize they have it until things are getting advanced. Warning signs of gum disease include:

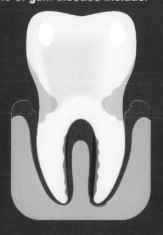

- Red, swollen, or tender gums
- A sore mouth
- Bleeding while brushing, flossing, or eating hard food
- Receding gums
- Changes in the way teeth "fit together" when biting

What Causes Gum Disease?

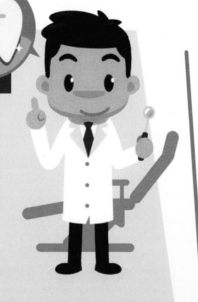

- Poor nutrition
- Failure to brush or floss teeth
- Smoking
- Medications
- Female hormone changes
- Underlying immune deficiencies (such as AIDS)
- Heredity
- Stress
- Aging
- Defective fillings or bridges
- Diabetes

PREMATURE BIRTHS HAVE BEEN LINKED TO GUM DISEASE.

Researchers have found that mothers with unhealthy gums are more likely to deliver premature or low birth weight babies. Hormonal changes triggered by contraceptives, pregnancy, or other reasons can all contribute to gum disease in women.

Smokers are 4x more likely to get advanced gum disease. If your parents had advanced gum disease, you are 12x more likely to host the bad bacteria that causes it.

Are Mouthwashes the Answer?

Mouthwashes kill bad bacteria. Some studies have even reported that mouthwashes can kill the COVID virus. Despite these good things, there are several reasons why mouthwashes are not a good way to fight gum disease:

- Many mouthwashes contain alcohol, leaving a dry mouth, which is highly detrimental in the war against bacteria.
- Mouthwashes touted for killing 99.9% of bacteria destroy the good as well as bad. This damages the microbiome in the mouth, limiting its ability to fight cavities, gingivitis and bad breath. This impaired microbiome is then passed down to the gut.
- Mouthwashes can make the mouth feel clean when it isn't, which encourages some to neglect daily dental routines such as brushing and flossing.
- Researchers have linked the decreased bacteria production caused by mouthwash use to lower nitrate production and increased risk of cardiovascular disease.
- The stabilizing agents used in many commercial mouthwashes, which are acidic, can cause tooth decay by eating away at tooth enamel.
- Many mouthwashes also include artificial food dyes, some of which have been identified as cancer causing agents.

BOTTOM LINE: Using commercial mouthwashes is like putting an unnecessary microbiome-disrupting antibiotic in your mouth.

Chemicals in Toothpastes

Most commercial toothpastes include harsh chemicals that aren't good for the teeth or gums. While these chemicals may make the mouth feel smooth or taste good, they aren't healthy overall. Some also destroy good bacteria. Ingredients to avoid include: aluminum hydroxide, aspartame, carrageenan, DEA (diethanolamine), flavorings, food coloring, formaldehyde releasing preservatives, parabens, potassium sorbate, propylene glycol, sodium benzoate, sodium lauryl sulfate, sodiumsaccharin, titanium dioxide, and triclosan.

MOUTHWASH INGREDIENTS TO AVOID: Alcohol, chlorine dioxide, chlorhexidine, cocamidopropylbetaine, parabens, Poloxamer 407, formaldehyde, and saccharin. If you would really like to use a mouthwash, try making your own. There are some healthy, homemade recipes on the Internet. As a bonus, you'll know what you're putting into your mouth!

Quick Tips to Improve Dental Health

Making improvements in diet is one of the very best ways to fight gum disease and improve dental health. Some dietary choices feed bad bacteria (e.g. sugar, junk foods, and processed foods) while others feed the good (e.g. a whole foods plant-based diet). Moving your choices in the right direction is a major step towards improving mouth health. In addition to making healthier diet choices, you can also help the "good guys" bacteria in your mouth by following the advice below:

- **Don't smoke.**
- **Brush twice daily for two minutes.**
- **Floss twice daily.**
- **Visit a dentist twice a year.**

Action Plan

→ Understand the direct link between the health of your mouth and your body, and take the steps necessary to improve and maintain a thriving set of good bacteria in your mouth.

→ If you find yourself in situations where you must wear masks for extended periods of time, do everything you can in other areas to promote good oral health.

→ Review the causes of gum disease and work to improve those you have control over.

→ Consider your daily dental care routine to see if there is room for improvement, and make the necessary changes.

→ Review the ingredients in any toothpaste, mouthwash, or other dental products you are using, and throw out those that are harmful.

→ If there is a toothache or infection in your mouth which you haven't been able to stop, visit a dentist ASAP. Taking pain killers while the infection persists allows bad bacteria to gain a stronger foothold in your body.

→ Visit the dentist two times per year whether you have a toothache or not. A good dental cleaning will remove any plaque (bacteria) buildup on your teeth and assist in your journey to a healthier mouth.

RECOVER YOUR JOY:
Powerful Steps You Can Take

Like the Spanish Flu of 1918, the COVID-19 pandemic took a huge toll on the health and psyches of many people, not to mention lives. In the midst of such social upheaval, restrictions, health challenges and sadness, it has been easy to lose our "joy." Yet somehow, though a tremendous hole has been left in our hearts by those we have lost, we must choose to "carry on." Though we take time to grieve, we cannot be glum forever. To do so would be draining not only for our health, but that of our children. And so, we must "recover our joy."

Stress Without Distress is Our Goal

Perhaps you have dreamed of a "stress-free" life. If so, you are not alone. However, as illustrated by the chart on this page:

- A stress-free life is actually a bad thing
- Without any stress at all, we lose our sense of purpose
- Productivity, happiness, and even our immune systems are diminished when "good stress" is missing from the life

At the same time, too much stress leads to:

- Distress
- Anxiety, panic, and/or anger
- Burnout and even breakdowns
- Higher cortisol levels
- Impaired immune system function

One key to recovering our joy is learning to manage stress without distress, which will open the door for productivity, happiness, and health to be at its peak.

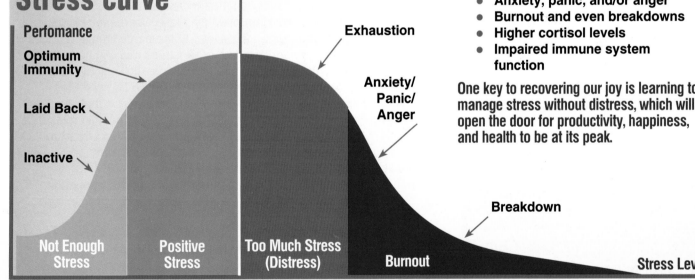

Stress curve

Perfomance

Optimum Immunity

Laid Back

Inactive

Exhaustion

Anxiety/ Panic/ Anger

Breakdown

Not Enough Stress

Positive Stress

Too Much Stress (Distress)

Burnout

Stress Level

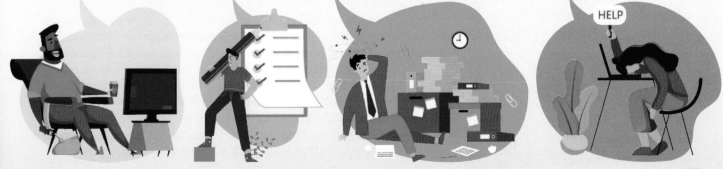

HELP

LAUGHTER: Still the Best Medicine

Back in 1875, a strait-laced gentleman by the name of George Vasey wrote a book vilifying laughter. In his tedious tome, Vasey opined that:

- Only "the depraved, the dissipated, and the criminal" were "addicted to uproarious mirth."
- Laughter was an idiotic, ugly, and vulgar habit reserved for empty-headed fools.
- By blocking the passage of air to the lungs, laughing not only distorted the face, but often led to fatalities.
- Sensible people would never be caught laughing, under any circumstances.

NOTE: While the Greek philosopher Chrysippus is said to have died by laughing at his own joke, this would be the exception, rather than the rule!

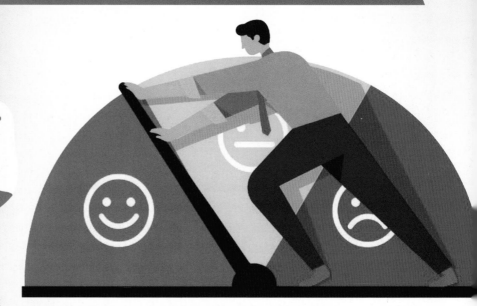

7 Ways to Laugh More

1. Get together with family or old friends and laugh about old pictures or times.

2. Learn to laugh at yourself and look for the humor in otherwise annoying situations.

3. Record a "Laughie" (a one minute audio of yourself chortling merrily), then giggle your way through it with others.

4. Join in a game night, karaoke night, or other fun social event.

5. Share a joke every day with others.

6. Spend more time with the funny people in your life.

7. Make a collection of things you find funny. Then, when you are feeling down, review your collection.

Fortunately, not all Victorians shared Vasey's derogatory view of the human habit of mirth. Indeed, the scientific evidence is firmly on the side of laughter as beneficial. Positive health results associated with laughter include:

- **Improved Blood Flow:** Researchers have found that, while stress reduces blood flow by 35%, laughter increases it by 22%. That's a 57% swing! This improved circulation increases oxygen and endorphin (feel-good hormone) levels. At the same time, it reduces levels of cortisol, epinephrine, and other stress causing hormones.
- **Unintentional Exercise:** When you laugh, your abdominal muscles expand and contract just as they would if you did some sit-ups (except you didn't have to do the work). How sweet is that!
- **Pain Reduction:** Scientists have linked laughter to muscle relaxation, which helps to break the pain-spasm cycle associated with chronic pain and muscle disorders. Laughter also releases endorphins, which are like natural pain killers to the body.
- **Reduced Blood Pressure:** The deep breathing that occurs during a good laugh dilates the blood vessels, resulting in a drop in blood pressure.
- **Boosted Immune System:** Laughter has been found to boost the "T cells" and neuropeptides that help the body to ward off disease. It also increases infection-fighting antibodies, immune-regulating cells, and cells that seek out and destroy viral and tumor cells.
- **Healthier Internal Organs:** The increased oxygen levels resulting from the deep breathing that occurs during laughter stimulates the brain, heart, lungs, and various muscles in the body. This stimulation increases cell regeneration and also improves overall organ health.
- **Calorie Burning:** Researchers from Vanderbilt University Medical Center found that, depending on body type, 10-15 minutes of deep belly laughing can burn 10-40 calories. For a 160-pound person, this would be about the same as walking 10 minutes on a treadmill at a rate of 2 miles per hour. (Perhaps you could double up the benefit, by reading a joke book while on the treadmill...)

Health Benefits of Strong Social Ties

Social connections are another powerful way to boost the immune system and retain sanity during pandemic times. In one landmark study, lack of social connection was seen as a greater detriment to health than obesity, smoking, and high blood pressure. That's what made the loss of social connection that resulted from quarantining, social distancing, and the general disruption of normal social structure so very costly in the fight against COVID-19. Ironically, some drastic steps taken to curb the spread of the virus resulted in immune-weakening side effects which made people more vulnerable to its spread. While there have been no perfect answers to this situation, it is up to all of us to realize the importance of social connection and maintain close ties to others even in difficult times. Evidence-based health benefits of strong social ties include:

- **Reduced blood pressure, heart rate, and stress hormone levels**
- **Lower rates of anxiety and depression**
- **Better emotion regulation skills**
- **Less inflammation throughout the body**
- **Faster and better recovery from illness and disease**

CORONAVIRUS DEATHS

ISOLATION

LONELINESS

ANXIETY

LOSS OF COMMUNITY

SOCIAL DISTANCING

DEPRESSION

SUICIDE

THE HAPPINESS-INDUCING IMMUNE-BOOSTING BENEFITS OF PLAY

While play comes naturally to youngsters, many adults see it as childish and a waste of time. Nothing could be further from the truth, however. Play, which is extremely beneficial to children in many ways, can also help adults through:

- **STRESS RELIEF:** As a fun activity, play releases the body's endorphins, a set of "feel good' chemicals that can promote an overall sense of well-being and even relieve pain.
- **IMPROVED BRAIN FUNCTION:** Fun activities that challenge the brain can improve brain function, stave off memory problems, and boost mood overall.
- **HEIGHTENED CREATIVITY:** Adults as well as children often learn best when they are feeling relaxed and playful. Play can also stimulate the imagination, which in turn boosts adaptation and problem-solving skills.
- **STRENGTHENED RELATIONSHIPS:** Shared laughter fosters compassion, empathy, intimacy, and trust. A playful state of mind is also great for soothing awkward situations, breaking the ice with strangers, and building new friendships. Play can also help heal emotional wounds, hurt and resentment.
- **BOOSTED ENERGY, VITALITY, AND DISEASE RESISTANCE:** Researchers have found enjoying a bit of playful "abandon" improves immune system function and resistance to disease.

Post-pandemic, one of the best steps we can take towards seeking to "recover the joy" in our lives is remembering how to play. To this end, there are a number of lessons we can learn from the animal world.

A merry heart doeth good like a medicine, but a broken spirit drieth the bones.
— Proverbs 17:22

When We Give, We Receive

Engaging in acts of service or kindness for others is one of the best ways to build and improve social ties. Researchers have found that acts of compassion and giving:

- **Create a sense of direction and purpose**
- **Are extremely beneficial to the "giver"**

While efforts to make the world a sunnier and happier place are a real connection and immune system booster, self-focus has been positively linked to immune-reducing stress.

BOTTOM LINE: When we help others, we are also helping ourselves!

More Examples of Play from the Animal Kingdom

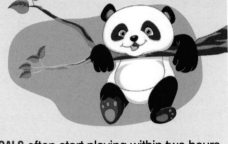
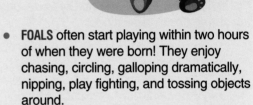

- **CATS** and kittens love to stalk, chase, pounce, swat, and bite each other — but it's all in good fun.

- **CROCODILES** love to slide down slippery slopes. They can also surf waves, and like to play with objects (like lilies floating in a pond).

- **PUPPIES** love to bounce, chase, growl, yip, and nibble. When a puppie "bows" this means they are being playful and not aggressive — a behavior which continues into adulthood.

- **DOLPHINS** love to jump, flip, somersault, blow bubble rings, and chase each other for the sheer joy of playing. Even older dolphins are very curious, and they love to make up their own games.

- To show that it wants to play, an **ELEPHANT** will cheerfully waggle its head and "dance." Young elephants often wiggle against each other and squirm on the ground. For their part, older elephants often let the young 'uns climb all over them.

- **FISH** love to leap playfully over objects like sticks, rocks, and turtles.

- **HERRING GULLS** like to play a game called "drop catch," where they drop clams and try to catch them before they land. Although herring gulls do eat clams, they don't usually eat the ones they play with.

- **FOALS** often start playing within two hours of when they were born! They enjoy chasing, circling, galloping dramatically, nipping, play fighting, and tossing objects around.

- **SEA OTTERS** love to slide, toss pebbles, wrestle, and play with their food before eating it.

- **BABY PANDA** bears love to climb trees, wrestle with each other, and zoom down slides. They also like to climb onto toys such as rocking horses.

- **YOUNG RAVENS** love to roll in the snow. They also like to fiddle with little things such as bottle caps, seashells, pebbles, and pieces of glass.

- From the moment they leave the pouch, **KANGAROOS** love to throw play punches at each other. They shake their heads to show they are playing. Adult kangaroos play fight too, except they often stand flat-footed and paw instead of throwing punches.

> *We don't stop playing because we grow old; we grow old because we stop playing.*
> — George Bernard Shaw

Action Plan

→ Take some time to consider the stress load in your life. Do you have manageable "good" stress? Or are you "distressed," overloaded, and facing burnout? If the latter is true, think of some baby steps you can take to change.

→ Think about how many times you have laughed in the last week. If you find yourself too burdened to laugh or smile, consider and implement some strategies to begin to find joy again.

→ Even if you are isolated, make efforts to keep social connections alive through phone calls, online groups, or video chats.

→ Schedule a "play night" once a week with family and/or friends.

BATTLE THE BULGE:
The Link Between Excess Pounds and COVID-19

Obesity nearly triples the risk of hospitalization from COVID-19. Excess pounds, which have been linked to impaired immune system function, increase pandemic-related risk for virtually anyone.

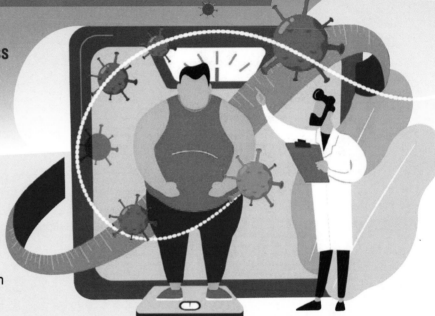

The higher the Body Mass Index (BMI), the higher the risk of COVID-related:

- Hospitalization
- ICU (Intensive Care Unit) Admission
- Mechanical ventilation
- Death

Obesity was not the only comorbidity rearing its ugly head during the pandemic. But it was a "big" one:

Percentage of hospitalized adult COVID-19 patients in the U.S. which had the following underlying medical conditions:

Hypertension	56%
Obesity	52%
Cardiovascular disease	32%
COPD	20%
Renal disease	14%
Asthma	3%

Preliminary hospitalizations as of April 18, 2020. U. S. adult prevalence latest available from CDC NHIS, NHANES or BRESS (2016-2018) Source: CDC

BEWARE OF... Well, Just Beware! THIN FOLKS ALERT!

- There's a "new kid" on the obesity block called osteosarcopenic obesity.
- People who lose bone density or are undermuscled have this condition.
- 30% of "visibly lean" people fit this description, making them metabolically obese.
- You can look thin and be metabolically obese at the same time.
- So looking thin doesn't automatically get you off the comorbidity hook.
- What we all need is metabolic health!

CHAPTER 20

THE GROWING PROBLEM OF OBESITY:
Startling Stats You Should Know

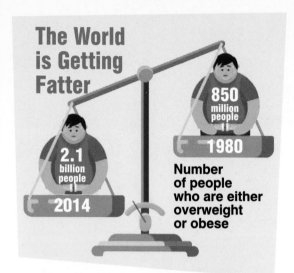

The World is Getting Fatter

850 million people
1980

2.1 billion people
2014

Number of people who are either overweight or obese

How to Know if You Are Overweight or Obese

CALCULATE YOUR BODY MASS INDEX (BMI) USING THIS FORMULA

BMI = weight (kg) / (height x height) (m)

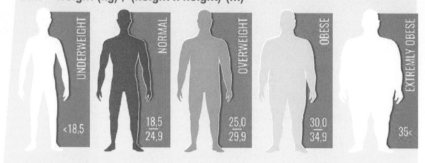

UNDERWEIGHT	NORMAL	OVERWEIGHT	OBESE	EXTREMELY OBESE
<18,5	18,5 24,9	25,0 29,9	30,0 34,9	35<

NOTE: Research is suggesting that people of Southeast Asian, Indian, African, Pacific Island, or Latin American descent should have a BMI of 23 or less. (BMI is a measure of body fat based on height and weight.)

OBESITY KILLS!
7 common diseases that result from obesity

1. Arthritis
2. Back pain
3. Cancer
4. Diabetes
5. Infertility
6. Stroke
7. Heart disease

Nearly 30%
of the world's population is obese or overweight

In many industrialized countries, the percentage of individuals who are either overweight or obese is more than 50%.

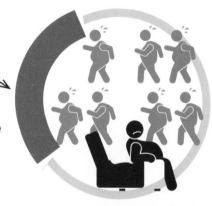

Why are excess pounds so harmful to immune system function?

BECAUSE THEY:

- Negatively impact ACE2 receptors (which are a protein found on many cell types). ACE2 receptors help regulate blood pressure, inflammation, and wound healing. In an overweight person, ACE2 receptors are out-of-whack before COVID ever strikes.

- Put the body into a state of chronic inflammation, which increases the presence of proinflammatory cytokines.

- Impair immunity through insulin and leptin resistance. The result is increased risk of disease and poor clinical outcomes when diseases such as COVID-19 strike.

In the middle of all this bad news, there is some good news!

OBESITY is Killing PREVENTABLE the WORLD

Top Tips for Dropping the Poundage

Tip №1: Fill Half Your Plate with Raw Veggies

While raw veggies might seem like a strange menu choice at breakfast, they provide important health benefits for a "turnaround diet." In addition to being low in calories and fat, raw veggies are an exceptional source of:

- The good gut bacteria which is so badly needed to improve overall health. Cooking tends to kill off the good bacteria, which is why raw veggies are best for this purpose.
- Fiber, vitamins, and health-promoting antioxidants.

NOTE: If you have a hard time with the veggies for breakfast, you can use fruit instead. Just be sure to use non-tropical fruits (such as berries) which have a lower glycemic Index. However, there really are a lot of benefits to eating a plate full of veggies in the morning.

Tip №2: Try the Nutritional Gastric Band

To lose weight quickly, try filling your tummy before a meal starts with the following remedy:

- TBSP glucomannan
- TBSP flax meal
- TBSP chia seed or psyllium husk
- CUP of water

Mix and drink immediately before a meal, as it thickens very quickly. Do this before each meal every day and watch the pounds drop off!

Tip №3: Curb Emotional Eating

Are you really hungry? Many people deal with emotional turmoil by turning to comfort foods. While such foods can be soothing, there are better ways to deal with emotions. (See the chapters in this book on peace and positive thoughts for some great ideas).

NOTE: When filling your plate, don't forget the "G-Bombs®" guide mentioned earlier in this book.

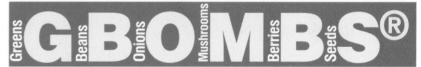

Greens **G** Beans **B** Onions **O** Mushrooms **M** Berries **B** Seeds **S** ®

As an added benefit, most options for the foods on the G-Bombs® list are low on the Glycemic Index scale.

Tip №4: Keep the Glycemic Index Value of Foods You Eat Below 55

The Glycemic Index (GI) is a system that ranks foods from 1 to 100 based on how quickly they raise blood sugar levels. Carbs with a high GI cause blood sugar levels to spike quickly, then crash. In contrast, low GI carbs are digested and released slowly for sustained energy. A lower GI diet can help with weight management by:

- Reducing insulin levels (which helps in fat burning)
- Helping you to feel full longer
- Fueling the body with sustained energy
- Improving mental performance

In addition to helping with weight management a low GI diet has been shown to be protective against heart disease, adult onset diabetes, macular degeneration, and some cancers.

IMPACT OF FOODS ON BLOOD SUGAR

High GI Foods

Low GI Foods

BLOOD GLUCOSE LEVELS

1 2

TIME / HOURS

Tip №5: Manage Your Mealtimes

In recent years, many people have discovered the benefits of Intermittent Fasting (IF). Although there are many "flavors" of IF, one of the simplest and most popular is simply to restrict the "eating window" each day. Setting mealtimes earlier in the day is also extremely beneficial to weight loss and better overall health, as outlined below:

Benefits of Intermittent Fasting
- A longer rest period for the digestive tract
- Better insulin regulation
- Improved microbiome (gut bacteria)
- More energy
- Faster weight loss
- Activated growth hormone
- Help in repairing a leaky gut

Benefits of Skipping Supper
- Bolstered growth hormone production
- Reduced risk of chronic disease such as diabetes and heart disease
- Increased stamina
- Reduction in elevated blood glucose and lipid levels

Tip №6: Get in Some Walking and Weight-bearing Exercise

Taking regular brisk walks, especially outdoors, remains one of the best ways to boost metabolism and improve overall health. Because muscle mass helps burn more calories, many people find some sort of weight-bearing exercise to also be beneficial in their personal battle against the bulge.

Tip №7: Stay Away from Free Fat

Low fat diets are never a good idea. Your brain needs fat to function well. In addition, it is the fat in food that provides the satiety needed to help you stop eating. Despite all the positive press that olive oil has received through the Mediterranean diet, the best diet for weight loss would NOT include free fats such as those in margarine, butter, and oil. For a therapeutic diet, the best places to get fat are olives, avocados, seeds, nuts, and other whole food sources.

Tip №9: Be Sure to Get Your Zzzzs

Lack of sleep can sabotage any weight loss program. Simply put, it is hard to exercise the self-control needed to stick with a program when the mind is exhausted. Deep sleep is when the body heals and repairs each night, which makes Zzz's even more critical to the process of removing excess fat in the tissues. We put sleep last on this list because it has already been covered in this book. However, addressing any shortage of sleep should be one of the first things you tackle in your weight loss efforts.

Tip №8: Drink Plenty of Water

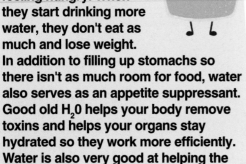

Many studies have shown that drinking water helps take off weight. Many people confuse dehydration with feeling hungry. When they start drinking more water, they don't eat as much and lose weight. In addition to filling up stomachs so there isn't as much room for food, water also serves as an appetite suppressant. Good old H_2O helps your body remove toxins and helps your organs stay hydrated so they work more efficiently. Water is also very good at helping the body to avoid storing fat.

Action Plan

→ Take stock of your personal health situation. Are you overweight, obese, or metabolically overweight (visually thin but undermuscled or suffering from bone loss)?

→ If the answer to any of the above questions is "yes," review this chapter and decide what you can do to get started on the journey towards better health.

→ Leap into action!

REST FROM DISTRESS

Finding Your Happy Place During Difficult Times

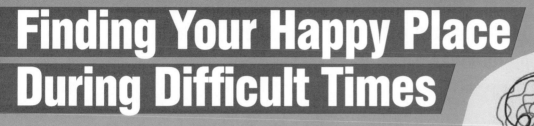

Adversity happens. We can't escape it. But we can handle it better. We can also stop creating our own. And we can be happy, even in difficult times. This chapter explores how.

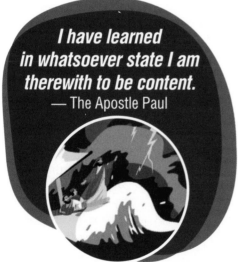

I have learned in whatsoever state I am therewith to be content.
— The Apostle Paul

The COVID-19 pandemic significantly increased the mental stress felt by many. In the U.S., the percentage of people experiencing symptoms of depression and anxiety surged to record highs (as illustrated by the chart below):

▮ **Before pandemic**   ▮ **After pandemic**

U.S. ADULTS REPORTING SYMPTOMS OF ANXIETY OR DEPRESSION

January – June 2019 ▮ 11%
December 2020 ▮ 40%

Source: Centers for Disease Control and Prevention.

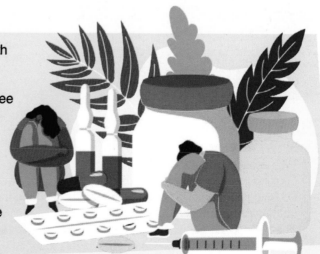

- Many of those struggling with depression and anxiety deal with those challenges through the use of prescription drugs.
- While psychiatric medications may be helpful or even be needed in some cases, challenges have arisen from the free use of psychiatric medications such as benzodiazepines, SSRIs, antipsychotic meds, stimulants, and others.
- Specifically, these medications create neurotransmitter imbalances and a resultant dependence.
- Fortunately, drugs are not the only way to cope with the stress of life.
- By making the most health-enhancing lifestyle choices, we can manage stress in ways that help us to optimize well-being and happiness.

TOOLS: In this book, we've already talked about some things you can do to optimize your immune system, as well as ways to better manage stress (e.g. positive thinking, social ties, and recovering your joy). In this chapter, we'd like to suggest a few more stress relief strategies to add to your mood-lifting, immune-building toolbox.

Correct "Thinking Errors"

- Without realizing it, many of us fall into thinking errors or "cognitive distortions" which end up causing immune-busting stress in our lives.

- Cognitive Behavioral Therapy (CBT) has helped many people change their thought patterns by taking responsibility for their own thinking.

- The idea that we can change how we act and feel by changing our thoughts is the basic concept behind CBT.

- Researchers have found that CBT is useful in many situations, including helping people to have better relationships, cope with grief, and reason through many of life's challenges.

- Even just reading a good book on CBT has been clinically proven to improve the mood and lift up the thinking. (For example, Feeling Good: The New Mood Therapy by Dr. David Burns has been clinically proven to have a positive impact on mental health for the majority of those who read it.)

- Following is a list of thinking errors (as proposed by Dr. Burns) that we all need to guard against.

THINKING ERROR №1:

Black & White (or Polarized) Thinking

- Everything is seen in absolutes (e.g. black and white, good and evil).
- Thinking is done in extremes. There is no middle ground.
- Because the truth or "reality" is usually somewhere in the middle, this thinking is most often unhelpful.
- Social media and online search engines feed polarized thinking by serving up results based on what people have searched for before. This tends to reinforce what they already think.
- This has contributed to a trend towards polarized (and even radical) thinking.
- To see clearly, we need to look at the big picture. While there are certainly moral absolutes, in many areas of life there should also be room for valid — but opposing — points of view.

THINKING ERROR №2: Sweeping Generalizations

- When people make sweeping generalizations, they draw important conclusions or assume there is a "rule of life" based on one experience. Watch out for the words "always" and "never."
- One negative event is seen by them as a never-ending pattern and justification for applying their negative conclusion "across the board."
- "My girlfriend broke up with me. I'm terrible at relationships and will never get married," is one example of a harmful generalization.
- Researchers have associated the thinking error of overgeneralization with anxiety disorders and PTSD.
- When pollsters take national surveys, they require a certain "sample size" before drawing conclusions. We need to do the same in our lives!

THINKING ERROR №3: Mental Filters

- We see what we set out to see.
- Looking through a mental filter is like looking at life through dirty glasses.
- Looking through an inaccurate mental filter can trigger or worsen both anxiety and depression.
- The feelings of hopelessness caused by such a negative perspective may become extreme enough to cause suicidal thoughts.

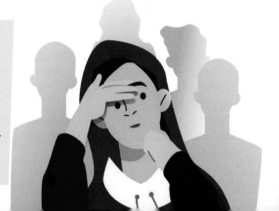

THINKING ERROR №4:
Explaining Away the Positive

- People who commit this thinking error actually do see the positives. But they just explain them away.
- For example, instead of recognizing that good outcomes result from skill, they might assume it was just a fluke.
- The trouble with this mental error is that it leads people to think they have no control over their circumstances.
- These negative beliefs reduce motivation and foster a sense of learned helplessness.

THINKING ERROR №6:
Fortune Teller Error

- People who commit this error think they know the future before the future arrives.
- One of the most common cognitive distortions, fortune teller error is linked to both anxiety and depression.

THINKING ERROR №5: Mind Reading

- Mind reading happens when people assume they know what others are thinking.
- The practice of mind reading, where people jump to conclusions based on what they assume the other is thinking, is the cause of many relationship problems.
- Even married couples who have been together for many years do not always know what the other is thinking!
- If in doubt at all about what another person is thinking, the best thing to do is ask!

THINKING ERROR №7:
Magnification or Minimization

- With this thinking error, people exaggerate the importance of something small or minimize the importance of something truly significant.
- The net result is that problems get blown way out of proportion while positive situations are ignored.
- Because this thinking error magnifies fears while minimizing adaptive behaviors, people with magnification or minimization challenges are often prone to panic attacks.
- The key to overcoming this distortion is to back up and see the big picture.

THINKING ERROR №8: Emotional Reasoning

- Because emotional reasoners take whatever they feel as the "gospel truth," they often rely on gut feelings to make major decisions.
- Emotional reasoners have trouble separating their feelings from the facts.
- While emotions are an important part of our thinking process, we also need to be aware of the facts!
- Emotional reasoning is the number one cause of laziness. "I don't feel like working, therefore I won't."

THINKING ERROR №9:
Labeling

- Labelers take one characteristic action of a person (even themselves) and apply it to the whole person. For example, if someone is rude one time, they are forever labeled as a jerk. The circumstances of the "jerkdom" don't matter and there is no forgiveness: once a "jerk," always a jerk.
- Labeling fuels and maintains negative emotions. It is very detrimental to relationships and can lead to negative behaviors.
- If you think you are dealing with a kind person who just made a mistake, the door is open to talk to them and work things out. Once you've labeled someone as a jerk or some other negative name, it becomes much harder to find solutions.

THINKING ERROR №10: Personalization

- People who take things that aren't really connected to them at all — personally — commit this thinking error.
- Examples of personalization include blaming yourself for things that aren't your fault or believing that you are being intentionally targeted or excluded when really you aren't.
- Researchers have linked personalization to feelings of inappropriate guilt.

Venting is Out, Forgiveness is In

- The Western World, and particularly the U.S., has been described by psychologist Dr. Martin Seligman as a "ventilationist society that deems it honest, just and even healthy to express our anger."
- While there are times when we need to communicate and even express our emotions, venting is problematic since anger tends to worsen when it is expressed.
- Road rage is a prime example of escalated feelings that, if handled in positive ways, would have saved lives.
- Researchers have shown that anger is detrimental to physical health. On the other hand, forgiveness has been shown to promote health by giving a sense of relief and even lowering blood pressure.

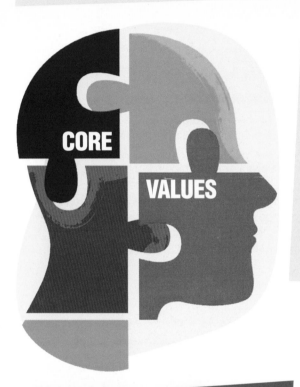

CORE VALUES

Make Peace with Yourself

- Going against one's conscience is one of the 10 "Hits" mentioned in the next chapter that contributes to immune-busting depression.
- When we proclaim one set of life values but live another, we create "cognitive dissonance" that puts us under a continual state of stress.
- For example, if we say our children are extremely important to us but spend little time with them, we are living one thing and doing another.
- Honestly considering our values, and whether we are living out our core beliefs, is one of the most important stress-relieving things we can do.
- If you aren't sure what you value the most in life, ask yourself "what do I love to talk about, think about, or spend time on?" The answers to those questions will show what you really value.

How to Re-think Your Core Values

- Make a short list of the life values you really wish to strive for.
- Make a second list showing how you spend most of your time.
- Compare those lists to see how they "match up."

HINT: When you love to do something, no one has to make or "motivate" you to do it. Surfers surf because they love surfing. Skiers ski because they love skiing. When we are "forced" to do something or require outside motivation, things don't end well. A great example is the millions of dieters who force themselves into unpleasant regimens to lose weight. When good health is a passion, things become so much simpler!

Action Plan

→ If you have navigated through the pandemic with the help of prescription drugs or self-medicated with alcohol, recreational drugs or some other diversion, consider how to replace those stress-management mechanisms with healthier habits.

→ Consider the list of 10 thinking errors in light of your own life. When you are honest with yourself, do you feel you have slipped into one or more of those errors? If so, try to "zoom out," see the big picture, and straighten out your thinking.

→ If you are struggling with anxiety or depression, or feel like you might have fallen into some thinking errors, consider reading a good book on Cognitive Behavioral Therapy. If you are really in trouble, please seek help immediately.

→ Think of some times you have "vented." Has the outcome usually been good? If not, consider how you could improve your response to challenging situations.

→ Follow the steps on this page under the heading "How to Re-think Your Core Values." If there is stress or dissonance in your life caused by a gap between what you believe and how you are living, make a plan for how to relieve that stress.

CHOOSE PEACE:
The Power of Hope to Help

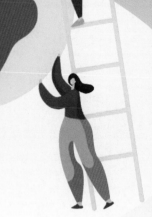

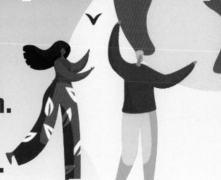

Many people don't realize that the way they think has a direct impact on their immune system. But it does — and the implications are truly profound.

STUDIES HAVE SHOWN THAT PEOPLE WITH MORE HOPE, OPTIMISM, AND POSITIVITY TEND TO HAVE:

- Stronger immune systems overall
- Higher levels of certain immune protective cells such as antibodies and T cells
- Lower blood pressure, triglycerides, and cholesterol than their more pessimistic peers

THOSE DWELLING ON THE SUNNIER SIDE OF LIFE ALSO TEND TO:

- Take better care of themselves through diet and exercise
- Trigger reward-related brain circuits through positive thoughts
- Have better coping skills, which reduces the harmful impact of stress on the body
- Have a lesser risk of premature death
- Live up to 15% longer than those with a more pessimistic outlook on life

WHY MOOD MATTERS —
Especially in Pandemic Times

Being stressed out, lonely, or depressed, actually increases your risk of "coming down" with COVID-19 or some other viral infection. It is actually a vicious cycle. The pandemic causes stress, which in turn raises our risk of infection, which then makes the pandemic worse. Quarantining and social distancing also contribute to loneliness, which makes people more likely to "catch" the very virus they are trying to avoid.

BOTTOM LINE: Lifting our spirits by cultivating hope should be a major priority, especially in difficult times.

In recent years, the study of the mind-immune system has developed into a new scientific field:

Psychoneuroimmunology (PNI)

Though the name might seem daunting, the meaning is really quite simple:

- Psycho refers to the mind
- Neuro refers to the brain
- Immunology refers to how the immune system works

Through PNI, scientists are discovering more and more ways that the brain impacts the immune system and overall wellness. This is actually very good news, since it gives us another very powerful weapon to implement in the fight against COVID-19 and other health threats.

6 WAYS TO BE A MORE HOPEFUL and Positive Person

Gonna be OK :)

Regardless of what you call it, we all know that hope, optimism, or positive thinking can be pretty good things. The real question is, how can we be more hopeful — especially if life has dealt us some pretty low blows. Any one of the following six strategies can get us started on the road to recovery:

1 Pep up your body language.

Remember — whatever you focus on, you feel. So refuse to pout. Stand tall with your head up and shoulders back, even if you don't feel like it. You may be surprised at the impact this one change can have on your mood!

2 Share a smile.

If that doesn't work, smile again. If someone else has no smile to give, bless them with one of yours.

3 Delete Your Inner Debbie Downer (or Negative Nate).

Negative people like to dwell on how bad they have it, sharing their list of woes to anyone who will listen. This can put a strain on relationships, plus make problems seem worse than they really are.

4 Specialize in Being Nice!

Pass out "pleases" and "thank-yous" with abandon. Try to catch others doing things right, and spend your time commending rather than criticizing. Feel free to apologize as needed and pay something forward whenever you can. If you haven't tried it before, you're likely to find that grace — and courteous behavior — are truly contagious!

6 Nix the Negative Words and Phrases.

Clear sweeping negative phrases and words (e.g. the "Horrible-Terrible-Awfuls") out of your vocabulary. Toning down our language, or modifying into more positive words, is a powerful way to lift off from "Grumpyland" into more sunshiny territory. Biggies to ban on the list of mood-slaying cliches include things like: "I suck," "you're so bad," and "how could you?"

5 Make a Gratitude List.

Write out a list of ten people, places, or things that you are super grateful for. Keep this list handy, and refer to it when you feel down.

NOTE: If someone dear to you has just passed or you've been through a traumatic event, it is normal to be sad. When faced with such "situational depression," it is important not to beat ourselves up. We need to work our way through whatever grief we encounter — plus understand that healing takes time.

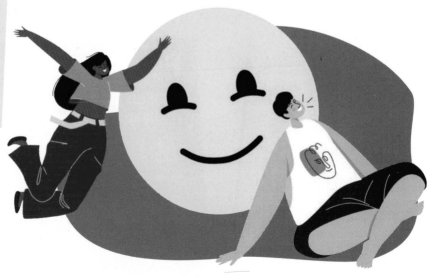

Understanding Why Depression Strikes

In our efforts to treat depression, it can be helpful to know the reasons behind the poor mood. Drs. Neil Nedley and Eddie Ramirez have documented that one evidence-based way to measure and even predict depression is through 10 "Hit" factors. If a person has four or more of these "Hits" in their life, they will be depressed. Furthermore, the more "Hits" sustained, the more depressed the person is likely to be. The 10 "Hit" categories that so often trigger depression are:

1. **GENETIC:** A family history of depression or suicide
2. **DEVELOPMENTAL:** Early puberty in girls, teenage depression, being raised in a non-traditional, abusive, or addiction-ridden home
3. **LIFESTYLE:** Lack of exercise, fresh air, or sunlight exposure
4. **POOR SLEEP:** Insomnia or sleep deprivation
5. **ADDICTIONS:** Alcohol, tobacco, caffeine (heavy users), recreational drugs, etc.
6. **NUTRITION:** An unhealthy diet or nutritional deficiencies
7. **TOXINS:** Including high levels of lead, mercury, arsenic, etc.
8. **SOCIAL STRESS:** Including the absence of social support, negative or stressful life events, low social class, being raised by grandparents, or having an immediate family member who struggles with addictions
9. **MEDICAL CONDITIONS:** Serious illnesses that require professional treatment
10. **FRONTAL LOBE:** Regularly going against one's conscience, or making lifestyle choices that negatively impact frontal lobe function (e.g. excessive TV viewing, gaming, sexual addictions, and gambling addictions)

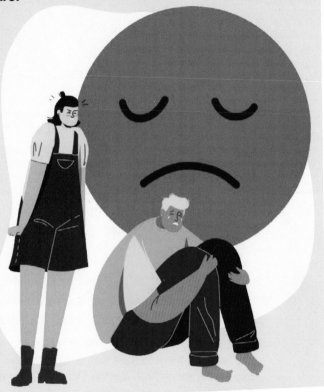

7 Blues-Busting Lifestyle Choices You Can Make

Many of the health-building strategies suggested in this book not only boost mood, but help to stave off depression. The following lifestyle therapies have been proven to fight the blues:

1. Adequate, restful sleep (at least 7 hours per night, but not more than 9)
2. Bright light therapy (sunshine or medical grade indoor lights can help)
3. Classical music therapy (beautiful, metered tunes such as Christian hymns or baroque music are best)
4. Daily spiritual exercise (such as Bible study or prayer)
5. Deep breathing exercises (especially outdoors or in a forest)
6. Regular physical exercise (outdoor exercise that raises the heart rate is best)
7. Hydrotherapy (hot and cold treatments are especially good at stimulating mood-enhancing blood flow to the frontal lobe)

RECOGNIZING "WHY" YOU FEEL DEPRESSED IS THE FIRST STEP TOWARD HEALING.

When an individual realizes that they have multiple "Hits" that are beyond their control (e.g. genetic, developmental, or an already existing medical condition) they can realize the importance of altering the "Hits" they do have control over.

Faith Matters

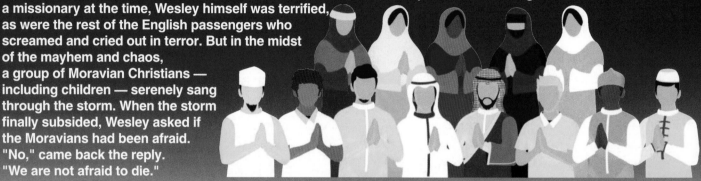

The great Protestant minister, John Wesley, was onboard a ship bound for America in 1735 when a terrible storm arose. At the height of the storm, waves broke over the ship, split the main sail in pieces, and poured in between the decks. To those on board, it seemed as if all hope was lost. Though a Christian and even a missionary at the time, Wesley himself was terrified, as were the rest of the English passengers who screamed and cried out in terror. But in the midst of the mayhem and chaos, a group of Moravian Christians — including children — serenely sang through the storm. When the storm finally subsided, Wesley asked if the Moravians had been afraid. "No," came back the reply. "We are not afraid to die."

 QUESTION: Why do some people find "peace in the storm" when others are terrified? This question has been asked for literally centuries on end. Why have some people calmly walked the plank, eyeballed a firing squad, gone "down with the ship," or even faced a pandemic — while others are frozen in fear?

 ANSWER: One important piece of the "calmness puzzle" that has received attention in recent years is the relationship between religion and resilience. A review of scientific studies on the impact of faith in hard times has revealed some fascinating facts. In one U.S. survey, researchers documented that:

- More than 40% of medical patients in some areas of the U.S. said that religion was the most important factor that enabled them to cope with illness. Another 50% in the same survey stated that their faith helped to a moderate or large degree. Only 10% of patients indicated that they received little or no comfort from their faith.
- In another study, scientists found that Bible-believing Christians were more optimistic than those from more liberal religious traditions.

IN CHAPTER 1 OF THIS BOOK, WE TALKED ABOUT HOW, DURING THE PLAGUES THAT DEVASTATED THE ROMAN EMPIRE, THE CHRISTIANS STAYED BEHIND TO TEND TO THE SICK WHILE THE PAGANS FLED IN FEAR. TODAY, SCIENTISTS ARE DOCUMENTING THAT A STRONG FAITH IN GOD IS A CALMING FACTOR THAT, IN ADDITION TO BOOSTING OUR POWER TO COPE, ACTUALLY HAS A POSITIVE EFFECT ON IMMUNE SYSTEM FUNCTION.

Action Plan

→ Review the ways (recommended in this chapter) to be a more hopeful and positive person. If you haven't been practicing those mood-boosting strategies in your life, decide which one(s) to try, and get started.

→ Consider the lifestyle choices on the same page as well, and try out one or more that you think might be helpful to you.

→ Re-read the list of "Hits" that trigger depression. Consider the ones you have control over, and how you can use those to reduce your risk of depression.

→ If you aren't already, try reading a Bible passage from Proverbs every day for a week. We also recommend looking up some of the many texts where the Bible uses the words "Fear not" or "Do not be afraid."

→ Try bringing your troubles to God. "Casting all your care upon Him, for He careth for you." (1 Peter 5:7)

CHAPTER 1 – STUDY HISTORY

- "Every Home a Sanitarium," Life & Health Magazine, May, 1919: Vol. 34.
- "Hutchinson Institution Makes a Record Combating Disease," Hutchinson Leader, December 13, 1918.
- A. B. Olsen, "How to Survive Influenza," Life & Health Magazine, May, 1919: Vol. 34.
- Abraham JP, et al. Using heat to kill SARS-CoV-2. Reviews in Medical Virology. 2020 Sep;30(5):e2115.
- American Public Health Association. Weapons Against Influenza. American Journal of Public Health. 1918 Oct;8(10):787-8.
- Fargey KM. The Deadliest enemy. Army History. 2019 Apr 1(111):24-39.
- Fears JR. The plague under Marcus Aurelius and the decline and fall of the Roman Empire. Infectious Disease Clinics. 2004 Mar 1;18(1):65-77.
- Franchimont P, et al. Hydrotherapy-mechanisms and indications. Pharmacology & therapeutics. 1983 Jan 1;20(1):79-93.
- Galli F, et al. Better prepare for the next one. Lifestyle lessons from the COVID-19 pandemic. PharmaNutrition. 2020 Jun;12:100193.
- Hobday RA, Cason JW. The open-air treatment of pandemic influenza. American journal of public health. 2009 Oct;99(S2):S236-42.
- Hobday RA. The open-air factor and infection control. Journal of Hospital Infection. 2019 Sep 1;103(1):e23-4.
- https://www.alaskapublic.org/2020/05/06/what-alaskans-learned-from-the-mother-of-all-pandemics-in-1918/
- https://www.tenement.org/the-flu-of-1918-sneeze-but-dont-scatter/
- Huremović D. Brief history of pandemics (pandemics throughout history). InPsychiatry of pandemics 2019 (pp. 7-35). Springer, Cham.
- Iddir M, et al. Strengthening the immune system and reducing inflammation and oxidative stress through diet and nutrition: considerations during the COVID-19 crisis. Nutrients. 2020 Jun;12(6):1562.
- Johnson NP, Mueller J. Updating the accounts: global mortality of the 1918-1920 "Spanish" influenza pandemic. Bulletin of the History of Medicine. 2002 Apr 1:105-15.
- Koch A, et al. system impacts of the European arrival and Great Dying in the Americas after 1492. Quaternary Science Reviews. 2019 Mar 1;207:13-36.
- L. E. Elliott, "The Value of Sanitarium Treatment in Respiratory Diseases," Life & Health Magazine, May, 1919: Vol. 34.
- Papagrigorakis MJ, et al. Typhoid fever epidemic in ancient Athens. InPaleomicrobiology 2008 (pp. 161-173). Springer, Berlin, Heidelberg.
- Petrofsky J, et al. Moist heat or dry heat for delayed onset muscle soreness. Journal of clinical medicine research. 2013 Dec;5(6):416.
- Philbrick KJ. Epidemic Smallpox, Roman Demography, and the Rapid Growth of Early Christianity, 160 CE to 310 CE (Doctoral dissertation, Columbia University).
- Robertson JS, Inglis SC. Prospects for controlling future pandemics of influenza. Virus research. 2011 Dec 1;162(1-2):39-46.
- Shanks GD, Brundage JF. Pathogenic responses among young adults during the 1918 influenza pandemic. Emerging infectious diseases. 2012 Feb;18(2):201.
- Stange N. Politics of Plague: Ancient Epidemics and Their Impact on Society.
- Sudre CH, et al. Attributes and predictors of long COVID. Nature Medicine. 2021 Apr;27(4):626-31.
- Talty S. The illustrious dead: the terrifying story of how typhus killed Napoleon's greatest army. Broadway Books; 2010.
- Wilton P. Spanish flu outdid WWI in number of lives claimed. CMAJ: Canadian Medical Association Journal. 1993 Jun 1;148(11):2036.

CHAPTER 2 – GO TO BED

- Abbasmanesh M, et al. Effect of sleep deprivation on mood and reaction time in the athletes and non-athletes. Rooyesh-e-Ravanshenasi Journal (RRJ). 2019 Nov 10;8(8):55-62.
- Abe Y, et al. Stress coping behaviors and sleep hygiene practices in a sample of Japanese adults with insomnia. Sleep and Biological Rhythms. 2011 Jan;9(1):35-45.
- Adam K, Oswald I. Sleep is for tissue restoration. Journal of the Royal College of Physicians of London. 1977 Jul;11(4):376.
- American Psychological Association. More Sleep Would Make Most Americans Happier, Healthier and Safer.
- Aton SJ, Herzog ED. Come together, right… now: synchronization of rhythms in a mammalian circadian clock. Neuron. 2005 Nov 23;48(4):531-4.
- Auld F, et al. Evidence for the efficacy of melatonin in the treatment of primary adult sleep disorders. Sleep Medicine Reviews. 2017 Aug 1;34:10-22.
- Besedovsky L, et al. Sleep and immune function. Pflügers Archiv-European Journal of Physiology. 2012 Jan;463(1):121-37.
- Bin Heyat MB, et al. Progress in Detection of Insomnia Sleep Disorder: A Comprehensive Review. Current Drug Targets. 2021 Apr 1;22(6):672-84.
- Bryant PA, et al. Sick and tired: does sleep have a vital role in the immune system?. Nature Reviews Immunology. 2004 Jun;4(6):457-67.
- Cairney SA, et al. Memory consolidation is linked to spindle-mediated information processing during sleep. Current Biology. 2018 Mar 19;28(6):948-54.
- Cappuccio FP, et al. Sleep duration and all-cause mortality: a systematic review and meta-analysis of prospective studies. Sleep. 2010 May 1;33(5):585-92.
- Chaput JP, et al. Sleep timing, sleep consistency, and health in adults: a systematic review. Applied Physiology, Nutrition, and Metabolism. 2020;45(10):S232-47.
- Chaput JP. Is sleep deprivation a contributor to obesity in children?. Eating and Weight Disorders-Studies on Anorexia, Bulimia and Obesity. 2016 Mar 1;21(1):5-11.
- Cho CH, et al. Exposure to dim artificial light at night increases REM sleep and awakenings in humans. Chronobiology international. 2016 Jan 2;33(1):117-23.
- Cohen S, et al. Sleep habits and susceptibility to the common cold. Archives of internal medicine. 2009 Jan 12;169(1):62-7.
- Cooper CB, et al. Sleep deprivation and obesity in adults: a brief narrative review. BMJ open sport & exercise medicine. 2018 Oct 1;4(1):e000392.
- Cuzzocrea S, Reiter RJ. Pharmacological actions of melatonin in acute and chronic inflammation. Current topics in medicinal chemistry. 2002 Feb 1;2(2):153-65.
- Douglas NJ, et al. Respiration during sleep in normal man. Thorax. 1982 Nov 1;37(11):840-4.
- Fogel RB, et al. The effect of sleep onset on upper airway muscle activity in patients with sleep apnoea versus controls. The Journal of physiology. 2005 Apr;564(2):549-62.
- Gallant AR, et al. The night-eating syndrome and obesity. Obesity reviews. 2012 Jun;13(6):528-36.
- Hanson JA, Huecker MR. Sleep Deprivation. StatPearls [Internet]. 2020 Oct 15.
- Hlaing EE. Relations between subjective sleep quality, sleep self-efficacy and cognitive performance in young and older adults. Southern Illinois University at Carbondale; 2011.
- https://www.cdc.gov/sleep/data_statistics.html
- Jagannath A, et al. The genetics of circadian rhythms, sleep and health. Human molecular genetics. 2017 Oct 1;26(R2):R128-38.
- Knutson KL, Van Cauter E. Associations between sleep loss and increased risk of obesity and diabetes. Annals of the New York Academy of Sciences. 2008;1129:287.
- Lan L, et al. Thermal environment and sleep quality: A review. Energy and Buildings. 2017 Aug 15;149:101-13.
- Lee H, et al. Effects of exercise with or without light exposure on sleep quality and hormone reponses. Journal of exercise nutrition & biochemistry. 2014 Sep;18(3):293.
- Lewis PA, et al. How memory replay in sleep boosts creative problem-solving. Trends in cognitive sciences. 2018 Jun 1;22(6):491-503.
- Li Y, et al. Relationship between stressful life events and sleep quality: rumination as a mediator and resilience as a moderator. Frontiers in psychiatry. 2019 May 27;10:348.
- Liao C, et al. Effects of Window Opening on the Bedroom Environment and resulting Sleep Quality. Science and Technology for the Built Environment. 2021 May 7(just-accepted):1-24.
- Liao Y, et al. Sleep quality in cigarette smokers and nonsmokers: findings from the general population in central China. BMC public health. 2019 Dec;19(1):1-9.
- Mallon L, et al. Relationship between insomnia, depression, and mortality: a 12-year follow-up of older adults in the community. International Psychogeriatrics. 2000 Sep 1;12(3):295.
- Mindell JA, et al. Implementation of a nightly bedtime routine: How quickly do things improve?. Infant Behavior and Development. 2017 Nov 1;49:220-7.
- Mullan BA. Sleep, stress and health: A commentary. Stress and Health. 2014 Dec;30(5):433-5.
- Nagendra RP, et al. Meditation and its regulatory role on sleep. Frontiers in Neurology. 2012 Apr 18;3:54.
- Nutt D, Wilson S, Paterson L. Sleep disorders as core symptoms of depression. Dialogues in clinical neuroscience. 2008 Sep;10(3):329.
- Park J, et al. Lifetime coffee consumption, pineal gland volume, and sleep quality in late life. Sleep. 2018 Oct;41(10):zsy127.
- Prather AA, et al. Behaviorally assessed sleep and susceptibility to the common old. Sleep. 2015 Sep 1;38(9):1353-9.
- Ritter SM, et al. Good morning creativity: task reactivation during sleep enhances beneficial effect of sleep on creative performance. Journal of sleep research. 2012 Dec;21(6):643-7.
- Roth T. Insomnia: definition, prevalence, etiology, and consequences. Journal of clinical sleep medicine. 2007 Aug 15;3(5 suppl):S7-10.
- Salari N, et al. Prevalence of stress, anxiety, depression among the general population during the COVID-19 pandemic: a systematic review and meta-analysis. Globalization and health. 2020 Dec;16(1):1-1.
- Segers A, Depoortere I. Circadian clocks in the digestive system. Nature Reviews Gastroenterology & Hepatology. 2021 Feb 2:1-3.
- Shin JE, Kim JK. How a good sleep predicts life satisfaction: The role of zero-sum beliefs about happiness. Frontiers in psychology. 2018 Aug 28;9:1589.
- Uthgenannt D, et al. Effects of sleep on the production of cytokines in humans. Psychosomatic Medicine. 1995 Mar 1;57(2):97-104.
- Vieira E, et al. Clock Genes, Inflammation and the Immune System—Implications for Diabetes, Obesity and Neurodegenerative Diseases. International Journal of Molecular Sciences. 2020 Jan;21(24):9743.
- Vitiello MV. Sleep, alcohol and alcohol abuse. Addiction Biology. 1997 Apr;2(2):151-8.
- Wagner U, et al. Emotional memory formation is enhanced across sleep intervals with high amounts of rapid eye movement sleep. Learning & memory. 2001 Mar 1;8(2):112-9.
- Walker MP, et al. Cognitive flexibility across the sleep-wake cycle: REM-sleep enhancement of anagram problem solving. Cognitive Brain Research. 2002 Nov 1;14(3):317-24.
- Wardle-Pinkston S, et al. Insomnia and cognitive performance: A systematic review and meta-analysis. Sleep medicine reviews. 2019 Dec 1;48:101205.
- Watson EJ, et al. Caffeine consumption and sleep quality in Australian adults. Nutrients. 2016 Aug;8(8):479.
- Yuan R, et al. The effect of sleep deprivation on coronary heart disease. Chinese Medical Sciences Journal. 2016 Dec 1;31(4):247-53.

CHAPTER 3 – RUN A FEVER

- Al-Nouri L, Basheer K. Mothers' perceptions of fever in children. J Trop Pediatr. 2006 Apr;52(2):113-6.
- Bain BJ. Structure and function of red and white blood cells. Med (United Kingdom). 2017;45(4):187-93.
- Casadevall A. Thermal Restriction as an Antimicrobial Function of Fever. PLoS Pathog. 2016 May;12(5):e1005577.
- Chapman A. Physicians, plagues and progress: the history of western medicine from antiquity to antibiotics. Lion Hudson Limited; 2016.
- Currents N. Fever and Thermal Therapy. 2020;83(April):4-6.
- Dong L, et al. Fever phobia: A comparison survey between caregivers in the inpatient ward and caregivers at the outpatient department in a children's hospital in China. BMC Pediatr. 2015;15(1):163.
- Evans SS, et al. Fever and the thermal regulation of immunity: The immune system feels the heat. Nat Rev Immunol. 2015/05/15. 2015 Jun;15(6):335-49.
- Greaney JL, et al. Sympathetic control of reflex cutaneous vasoconstriction in human aging. J Appl Physiol. 2015/08/13. 2015 Oct;119(7):771-82.
- Haghayegh S, et al. Before-bedtime passive body heating by warm shower or bath to improve sleep: A systematic review and meta-analysis. Sleep Med Rev. 2019;46:124-35.
- Haman F, Blondin DP. Shivering thermogenesis in humans: Origin, contribution and metabolic requirement. Temperature. 2017 May;4(3):217-26.
- Harvard T. Medicine and Cosmology in Classical Greece : First Principles in Early Greek Medicine. 2016;
- Hasebe Y. Effects of hot compress treatment with a hot water bottle on physiological parameters and subjective sensations in healthy women. Japan J Nurs Sci. 2005;2(2):107-14.
- Jackson SW. Galen—on mental disorders. Journal of the History of the Behavioral Sciences. 1969 Oct;5(4):365-84.
- Kluger MJ. 4. The Adaptive Value of Fever. In: Fever: Its Biology, Evolution, and Function. Princeton University Press; 2015. p. 129-66.
- Lack LC, et al. The relationship between insomnia and body temperatures. Sleep Med Rev. 2008 Aug;12(4):307-17.
- Laukkanen JA, et al. Cardiovascular and Other Health Benefits of Sauna Bathing: A Review of the Evidence. Mayo Clin Proc. 2018;93(8):1111-21.
- Lee SY, et al. Oncological hyperthermia: The correct dosing in clinical applications. Int J Oncol. 2018/11/23. 2019 Feb;54(2):627-43.
- Lin F ching, Young HA. Interferons: Success in anti-viral immunotherapy. Cytokine Growth Factor Rev. 2014/07/29. 2014 Aug;25(4):369-76.
- Ludwig J, McWhinnie H. Antipyretic drugs in patients with fever and infection: Literature review. Br J Nurs. 2019 May;28(10):610-8.
- Murin CD, et al. Antibody responses to viral infections: a structural perspective across three different enveloped viruses. Nat Microbiol. 2019/03/18. 2019 May;4(5):734-47.
- Nicholson LB. The immune system. Essays Biochem. 2016 Oct;60(3):275-301.
- Nyce J. Alert to US physicians: DHEA, widely used as an OTC androgen supplement, may exacerbate COVID-19. Endocr Relat Cancer. 2021;28(2):R47-53.
- Ogoina D. Fever, fever patterns and diseases called "fever" - A review. J Infect Public Health. 2011;4(3):108-24.
- Papaioannou TG, et al. Heat therapy: an ancient concept re-examined in the era of advanced biomedical technologies. J Physiol. 2016 Dec;594(23):7141-2.
- Plaza JJG, et al. Role of metabolism during viral infections, and crosstalk with the innate immune system. Intractable Rare Dis Res. 2016 May;5(2):90-6.
- Prow NA, et al. Lower temperatures reduce type I interferon activity and promote alphaviral arthritis. PLoS Pathog. 2017 Dec;13(12):e1006788.
- Purssell E. Treatment of fever and over-the-counter medicines. Arch Dis Child. 2007/05/23. 2007 Oct;92(10):900-1.
- Rather IA, et al. Self-medication and antibiotic resistance: Crisis, current challenges, and prevention. Saudi J Biol Sci. 2017/01/09. 2017 May;24(4):808-12.
- Ray JJ, Schulman CI. Fever: Suppress or let it ride? J Thorac Dis. 2015 Dec;7(12):E633-6.
- Richmond VL, et al. Prediction of Core Body Temperature from Multiple Variables. Ann Occup Hyg. 2014 Nov;59(9):1168-78.
- Rotz PD. Winner of the Southern African historical society's student essay prize in 2015: Sweetness and fever? Sugar production, aedes aegypti, and dengue fever in Natal, South Africa, 1926-1927. South African Hist J. 2016 Jul;68(3):286-303.
- Sarkar D, et al. Alcohol and the immune system. Alcohol Res Curr Rev. 2015;37(2):153-5.
- Tansey EA, Johnson CD. Recent advances in thermoregulation. Adv Physiol Educ. 2015 Sep;39(1):139-48.
- Tsay CJ. Julius Wagner-Jauregg and the legacy of malarial therapy for the treatment of general paresis of the insane. Yale J Biol Med. 2013 Jun;86(2):245-54.
- Weiner DB. Philippe Pinel's "Memoir on Madness" of December 11, 1794: A fundamental text of modern psychiatry. Am J Psychiatry. 1992 Jun;149(6):725-32.
- Woesner1 ME. What is old is new again: The use of whole-body hyperthermia for depression recalls the medicinal uses of hyperthermia, fever therapy, and hydrotherapy. Curr Neurobiol [Internet]. 2019;10(2):56-66.
- Yagawa Y, et al. Cancer immunity and therapy using hyperthermia with immunotherapy, radiotherapy, chemotherapy, and surgery. J Cancer Metastasis Treat. 2017;3(10):218.
- Zhao ZD, et al. A hypothalamic circuit that controls body temperature. Proc Natl Acad Sci U S A. 2017 Feb;114(8):2042-7.

CHAPTER 4 – STEAM • SOAK • DETOX

- Bender T, et al. Hydrotherapy, balneotherapy, and spa treatment in pain management. Rheumatology international. 2005 Apr 1;25(3):220-4.
- Brenner IK, et al. Immune changes in humans during cold exposure: effects of prior heating and exercise. Journal of Applied Physiology. 1999 Aug 1.
- Church JM. Warm water irrigation for dealing with spasm during colonoscopy: simple, inexpensive, and effective. Gastrointestinal endoscopy. 2002 Nov 1;56(5):672-4.
- Coudevylle GR, et al. Impact of Cold Water Intake on Environmental Perceptions, Affect, and Attention Depends on Climate Condition. The American Journal of Psychology. 2020 Jul 1;133(2):205-19.
- Deaux E, Engstrom R. The temperature of ingested water: Its effect on body temperature. Physiological Psychology. 1973 Jun;1(2):152-4.
- Dubnov-Raz G, et al. Influence of water drinking on resting energy expenditure in overweight children. International journal of obesity. 2011 Oct;35(10):1295-300.
- https://finland.fi/life-society/bare-facts-of-the-sauna (This is Finland: Ministry of Foreign Affairs for Finland)
- https://sauna.fi/saunatietoa/ (Finnish Sauna Society)
- Iiyama J, et al. Effects of single low-temperature sauna bathing in patients with severe motor and intellectual disabilities. International journal of biometeorology. 2008 Jul;52(6):431-7.
- Kauppinen K. Sauna, shower, and ice water immersion. Physiological responses to brief exposures to heat, cool, and cold. Part II. Circulation. Arctic medical research. 1989 Apr 1;48(2):64-74.
- Kawahara Y, et al. Effects of bath water and bathroom temperatures on human thermoregulatory function and thermal perception during half-body bathing in winter. InElsevier Ergonomics Book Series 2005 Jan 1 (Vol. 3, pp. 171-176). Elsevier.
- Lee EC, et al. Interleukin-6 responses to water immersion therapy after acute exercise heat stress: a pilot investigation. Journal of athletic training. 2012;47(6):655-63.
- Liao S, von der Weid PY. Lymphatic system: an active pathway for immune protection. InSeminars in cell & developmental biology 2015 Feb 1 (Vol. 38, pp. 83-89). Academic Press.
- Liikkanen LA, Laukkanen JA. Sauna bathing frequency in Finland and the impact of COVID-19. Complementary Therapies in Medicine. 2021 Jan 1;56:102594.
- Moore Jr JE, Bertram CD. Lymphatic system flows. Annual review of fluid mechanics. 2018 Jan 5;50:459-82.
- Mooventhan A, Nivethitha L. Scientific evidence-based effects of hydrotherapy on various systems of the body. North American journal of medical sciences. 2014 May;6(5):199.
- Moss GA. Water and health: a forgotten connection?. Perspectives in public health. 2010 Sep;130(5):227-32.
- Naumann J, Sadaghiani C. Therapeutic benefit of balneotherapy and hydrotherapy in the management of fibromyalgia syndrome: a qualitative systematic review and meta-analysis of randomized controlled trials. Arthritis research & therapy. 2014 Aug;16(4):1-3.
- Petrofsky JS, et al. The effect of the moisture content of a local heat source on the blood flow response of the skin. Archives of dermatological research. 2009 Sep;301(8):581-5.
- Saketkhoo K, et al. Effects of drinking hot water, cold water, and chicken soup on nasal mucus velocity and nasal airflow resistance. Chest. 1978 Oct 1;74(4):408-10.
- Song CW, et al. Effects of temperature on blood circulation measured with the laser Doppler method. International Journal of Radiation Oncology* Biology* Physics. 1989 Nov 1;17(5):1041-7.
- Soto-Quijano DA, Grabois M. Hydrotherapy. In Pain Management 2007 Jan 1 (pp. 1043-1051). WB Saunders.
- Tochihara Y, Ohnaka T. Environmental Ergonomics-The Ergonomics of Human Comfort, Health, and Performance in the Thermal Environment. Elsevier; 2005 Apr 2.
- Van der Sluijs E, Slot DE, et al. The effect of water on morning bad breath: a randomized clinical trial. International journal of dental hygiene. 2016 May;14(2):124-34.
- Weston M, et al. Changes in local blood volume during cold gel pack application to traumatized ankles. Journal of Orthopaedic & Sports Physical Therapy. 1994 Apr;19(4):197-9.
- Yeung SS, et al. Effects of cold water immersion on muscle oxygenation during repeated bouts of fatiguing exercise: a randomized controlled study. Medicine. 2016 Jan;95(1).

CHAPTER 5 – BREATHE TO HEAL

- Alexander DD, et al. Air ions and respiratory function outcomes: A comprehensive review. Vol. 12, Journal of Negative Results in BioMedicine. 2013.
- Berman MG, et al. The cognitive benefits of interacting with nature. Psychological science. 2008 Dec;19(12):1207-12.
- Chevalier G, et al. Earthing: Health implications of reconnecting the human body to the Earth's surface electrons. J Environ Public Health. 2012;2012.
- Craig JM, et al. Natural environments, nature relatedness and the ecological theater: connecting satellites and sequencing to shinrin-yoku. Journal of physiological anthropology. 2016 Dec;35(1):1-0.Ewert A, Chang Y. Levels of Nature and Stress Response. Behav Sci (Basel).

REFERENCES

- Du S, et al. Laser guided ionic wind. Vol. 8, Scientific Reports. 2018.
- Engemann K, et al. Residential green space in childhood is associated with lower risk of psychiatric disorders from adolescence into adulthood. Proceedings of the national academy of sciences. 2019 Mar 12;116(11):5188-93.
- Franco LS, et al. A review of the benefits of nature experiences: more than meets the eye. International journal of environmental research and public health. 2017 Aug;14(8):864.
- Furuyashiki A, et al. A comparative study of the physiological and psychological effects of forest bathing (Shinrin-yoku) on working age people with and without depressive tendencies. Environmental health and preventive medicine. 2019 Dec;24(1):1-1.
- Grafetstätter C, et al. Does waterfall aerosol influence mucosal immunity and chronic stress? A randomized controlled clinical trial. Vol. 36, Journal of Physiological Anthropology. 2017.
- Hobday RA, Cason JW. The open-air treatment of pandemic influenza. American journal of public health. 2009 Oct;99(S2):S236-42.
- Hobday RA, Dancer SJ. Roles of sunlight and natural ventilation for controlling infection: historical and current perspectives. Journal of hospital infection. 2013 Aug 1;84(4):271-82.
- Jiang SY, et al. Negative air ions and their effects on human health and air quality improvement. International journal of molecular sciences. 2018 Oct;19(10):2966.
- Kuo M. How might contact with nature promote human health? Promising mechanisms and a possible central pathway. Frontiers in psychology. 2015 Aug 25;6:1093.
- Lazzerini F, et al. Progress of negative air ions in health tourism environments applications. Bol Soc Española Hidrol Medica. 2018;33(1):27-46.
- Li Q, et al. A forest bathing trip increases human natural killer activity and expression of anti-cancer proteins in female subjects. J Biol Regul Homeost Agents. 2008 Jan 1;22(1):45-55.
- Li Q, et al. Effects of forest bathing on cardiovascular and metabolic parameters in middle-aged males. Evidence-Based Complementary and Alternative Medicine. 2016 Jan 1;2016.
- Li Q, et al. Forest bathing enhances human natural killer activity and expression of anti-cancer proteins. International journal of immunopathology and pharmacology. 2007 Apr;20(2_suppl):3-8.
- Li Q, et al. Phytoncides (wood essential oils) induce human natural killer cell activity. Immunopharmacology and immunotoxicology. 2006 Jan 1;28(2):319-33.
- Lobo V, et al. Free radicals, antioxidants and functional foods: Impact on human health. Vol. 4, Pharmacognosy Reviews. 2010. p. 118-26.
- Mann D. Negative Ions Create Positive Vibes [Internet]. 2003. Available from: https://www.webmd.com/balance/features/negative-ions-create-positive-vibes#1
- Margaret M, et al. Shinrin-Yoku (Forest Bathing) and Nature Therapy: A State-of-the-Art Review.
- Morita E, et al. A before and after comparison of the effects of forest walking on the sleep of a community-based sample of people with sleep complaints. BioPsychoSocial medicine. 2011 Dec;5(1):1-7.
- Park BJ, et al. The physiological effects of Shinrin-yoku (taking in the forest atmosphere or forest bathing): evidence from field experiments in 24 forests across Japan. Environmental health and preventive medicine. 2010 Jan;15(1):18-26.
- Perez V, et al. Air ions and mood outcomes: A review and meta-analysis. Vol. 13, BMC Psychiatry. 2013.
- Pino O, La Ragione F. There's something in the air: Empirical evidence for the effects of negative air ions (NAI) on psychophysiological state and performance. Research in Psychology and Behavioral Sciences. 2013;1(4):48-53.
- Suzuki S, et al. Effects of negative air ions on activity of neural substrates involved in autonomic regulation in rats. International journal of biometeorology. 2008 Jul;52(6):481-9.
- US Environmental Protection Agency. Report to Congress on indoor air quality, volume II: assessment and control of indoor air pollution. Technical Report EPA/400/1-89/001C. 1989.
- Wang H, et al. Study on the change of negative air ion concentration and its influencing factors at different spatio-temporal scales. Vol. 23, Global Ecology and Conservation. 2020.
- Watanabe I, et al. Physical effects of negative air ions in a wet sauna. Vol. 40, International Journal of Biometeorology. 1997. p. 107-12.
- Wiszniewski A, et al. Effects of Air-Ions on Human Circulatory Indicators. Polish Journal of Environmental Studies. 2014 Mar 1;23(2).
- Yau KK, Loke AY. Effects of forest bathing on pre-hypertensive and hypertensive adults: a review of the literature. Environmental health and preventive medicine. 2020 Dec;25(1):1-7.
- Zeng C, et al. Benefits of a three-day bamboo forest therapy session on the physiological responses of university students. International journal of environmental research and public health. 2020 Jan;17(9):3238.
- Zhu SX, et al. Comprehensive Evaluation of Healthcare Benefits of Different Forest Types: A Case Study in Shimen National Forest Park, China. Forests. 2021 Feb;12(2):207.

CHAPTER 6 – GUARD YOUR NOSE

- Adams SH, et al. Medical vulnerability of young adults to severe COVID-19 illness–data from the National Health Interview Survey. Journal of Adolescent Health. 2020 Sep 1;67(3):362-8.
- Bartley J, McGlashan SR. Does milk increase mucus production?. Medical hypotheses. 2010 Apr 1;74(4):732-4.
- Braun SR. Respiratory rate and pattern. Clinical Methods: The History, Physical, and Laboratory Examinations. 3rd edition. 1990.
- Brett L, et al. Clinical course and prediction of survival in ideopathic pulmonary fibrosis. Am J Respir Crit Care Med. 2011;183:431-40.
- Brinkman JE, Toro F. Physiology, respiratory drive.[Updated 2020 May 24]. StatPearls [Internet]. Treasure Island (FL): StatPearls Publishing. 2020.
- Butler BD. Hills BA. The lung as a filter for microbubbles. J Appl Physiol. 1979;47:537-43.
- Cao Y, et al. Environmental pollutants damage airway epithelial cell cilia: Implications for the prevention of obstructive lung diseases. Thoracic cancer. 2020 Mar;11(3):505-10.
- Carey RM, Lee RJ. Taste receptors in upper airway innate immunity. Nutrients. 2019 Sep;11(9):2017.
- Castriotta RJ, et al. Workshop on idiopathic pulmonary fibrosis in older adults. Chest. 2010 Sep 1;138(3):693-703.
- Crisan-Dabija R, et al. "A Chain Only as Strong as Its Weakest Link": An Up-to-Date Literature Review on the Bidirectional Interaction of Pulmonary Fibrosis and COVID-19. Journal of Proteome Research. 2020 Sep 4;19(11):4327-38.
- Dhand R, Li J. Coughs and sneezes: their role in transmission of respiratory viral infections, including SARS-CoV-2. American journal of respiratory and critical care medicine. 2020 Sep 1;202(5):651-9.
- Dixon AE, Peters U. The effect of obesity on lung function. Expert Rev Respir Med 2018; 12: 755-67.
- Fan C, et al. Alterations in Oral-Nasal-Pharyngeal Microbiota and Salivary Proteins in Mouth-Breathing Children. Frontiers in Microbiology. 2020 Oct 9;11:2472.
- García-Arroyo FE, et al. Rehydration with soft drink-like beverages exacerbates dehydration and worsens dehydration-associated renal injury. American Journal of Physiology-Regulatory, Integrative and Comparative Physiology. 2016 Jul 1.
- Ghisa M, et al. Idiopathic pulmonary fibrosis and GERD: links and risks. Therapeutics and clinical risk management. 2019;15:1081.
- Gilroy Jr RJ, et al. Respiratory mechanical effects of abdominal distension. Journal of Applied Physiology. 1985 Jun 1;58(6):1997-2003.
- Gransee HM, et al. Respiratory muscle plasticity. Comprehensive Physiology. 2011 Jan 17;2(2):1441-62.
- Hasler WL. Gas and bloating. Gastroenterol Hepatol. 2006;2(9):654-62.
- Hassan AO, Feldmann F, Zhao H, Curiel DT, Okumura A, Tang-Huau TL, Case JB, Meade-White K, Callison J, Chen RE, Lovaglio J. A single intranasal dose of chimpanzee adenovirus-vectored vaccine protects against SARS-CoV-2 infection in rhesus macaques. Cell Reports Medicine. 2021 Apr 20;2(4):100230.
- Hsia CC, et al. Lung structure and the intrinsic challenges of gas exchange. Comprehensive physiology. 2011 Jan 17;6(2):827-95.
- https://www.lung.org/blog/how-your-lungs-work (American Lung Association)
- Janeway CA Jr, et al. Immunobiology: The Immune System in Health and Disease. 5th edition. New York: Garland Science; 2001. The mucosal immune system.
- Joseph D, et al. Non-respiratory functions of the lung. Continuing Education in Anaesthesia, Critical Care & Pain. 2013 Jun 1;13(3):98-102.
- Joyner MJ, Casey DP. Regulation of increased blood flow (hyperemia) to muscles during exercise: a hierarchy of competing physiological needs. Physiological reviews. 2015 Apr 1.
- Karwowska M, Kononiuk A. Nitrates/nitrites in food–Risk for nitrosative stress and benefits. Antioxidants. 2020 Mar;9(3):241.
- Knowles MR, Boucher RC. Mucus clearance as a primary innate defense mechanism for mammalian airways. The Journal of clinical investigation. 2002 Mar 1;109(5):571-7.
- Kubba S. Indoor Environmental Quality (IEQ). LEED v4 Practices, Certification, and Accreditation Handbook. 2016:303.
- Lee JS, et al. Does chronic microaspiration cause idiopathic pulmonary fibrosis?. The American journal of medicine. 2010 Apr 1;123(4):304-11.
- Lee JS, et al. Gastroesophageal reflux therapy is associated with longer survival in patients with idiopathic pulmonary fibrosis. American journal of respiratory and critical care medicine. 2011 Dec 15;184(12):1390-4.
- Lee RJ, Cohen NA. Taste receptors in innate immunity. Cellular and molecular life sciences. 2015 Jan;72(2):217-36.
- Magder S. Heart-Lung interaction in spontaneous breathing subjects: the basics. Annals of translational medicine. 2018 Sep;6(18).
- Pilette C, et al. Lung mucosal immunity: immunoglobulin-A revisited. European Respiratory Journal. 2001 Sep 1;18(3):571-88.
- Ra SH, et al. Upper respiratory viral load in asymptomatic individuals and mildly symptomatic patients with SARS-CoV-2 infection. Thorax. 2021 Jan 1;76(1):61-3.
- Randell SH, Boucher RC. Effective mucus clearance is essential for respiratory health. American journal of respiratory cell and molecular biology. 2006 Jul;35(1):20-8.
- Rhoades R, Tanner GA, editors. Medical physiology. Boston (MA): Little, Brown; 1995 Jan.
- Schwab JA, Zenkel M. Filtration of particulates in the human nose. The Laryngoscope. 1998 Jan;108(1):120-4.
- Scoditti E, et al. Role of diet in chronic obstructive pulmonary disease prevention and treatment. Nutrients. 2019 Jun;11(6):1357.
- Sharma RK, et al. Distribution of gingival inflammation in mouth breathing patients: an observational pilot study. Journal of Dentistry Indonesia. 2016;23(2):28-32.
- Spagnolo P, et al. The management of patients with idiopathic pulmonary fibrosis. Frontiers in medicine. 2018 Jul 2;5:148.
- Stickel S, et al. The practical management of fluid retention in adults with right heart failure due to pulmonary arterial hypertension. European Heart Journal Supplements. 2019 Dec 1;21(Supplement_K):K46-53.
- Subramanian CR, Triadafilopoulos G. Refractory gastroesophageal reflux disease. Gastroenterology report. 2015 Feb 1;3(1):41-53.
- Walser T, et al. Smoking and lung cancer: the role of inflammation. Proceedings of the American Thoracic Society. 2008 Dec 1;5(8):811-5.
- Weupe M, et al. Moving Mucus Matters for Lung Health. Front. Young Minds. (2019) 7:106.
- Wipfli HL, Samet JM. Second-hand smoke's worldwide disease toll. Lancet (London, England). 2010 Nov 25;377(9760):101-2.

CHAPTER 7 – HEAL YOUR GUT

- Blaser MJ, Dominguez-Bello MG. The human microbiome before birth. Cell host & microbe. 2016 Nov 9;20(5):558-60.
- Breit S, et al. Vagus nerve as modulator of the brain-gut axis in psychiatric and inflammatory disorders. Front Psychiatry. 2018 Mar;9(MAR):44.
- Davis CD. The gut microbiome and its role in obesity. Nutr Today. 2016;51(4):167-74.
- Derrien M, et al. The Gut Microbiota in the First Decade of Life. Trends Microbiol. 2019 Dec;27(12):997-1010.
- Dill-McFarland KA, et al. Close social relationships correlate with human gut microbiota composition. Sci Rep. 2019 Jan;9(1):703.
- Gagliardi A, et al. Rebuilding the gut microbiota ecosystem. Vol. 15, International Journal of Environmental Research and Public Health. 2018.
- Galland L. The gut microbiome and the brain. J Med Food. 2014 Dec;17(12):1261-72.
- Goldschmidt BV. Updated For 2018 : The Dirty Dozen And Clean 15 Fruits And Vegetables. 2018;1-8.
- Jenkins TA, et al. Influence of tryptophan and serotonin on mood and cognition with a possible role of the gut-brain axis. Nutrients. 2016 Jan;8(1).
- Kim JY, et al. The human gut archaeome: Identification of diverse haloarchaea in Korean subjects. Microbiome. 2020;8(1):114.
- Korpela K, et al. Selective maternal seeding and environment shape the human gut microbiome. Genome Res. 2018 Apr;28(4):561-8.
- Lacy BE, Spiegel B. Introduction to the Gut Microbiome Special Issue. Am J Gastroenterol. 2019;114(7):1013.
- Lam YY, et al. Are the gut bacteria telling us to eat or not to eat? Reviewing the role of gut microbiota in the etiology, disease progression and treatment of eating disorders. Nutrients. 2017 Jun;9(6):602.
- Lawrence K, Hyde J. Microbiome restoration diet improves digestion, cognition and physical and emotional wellbeing. PLoS One. 2017 Jun;12(6):e01790
- Lozupone CA, et al. Diversity, stability and resilience of the human gut microbiota. Nature. 2012 Sep;489(7415):220-30.
- Mills S, et al. Movers and shakers: Influence of bacteriophages in shaping the mammalian gut microbiota. Gut Microbes. 2013;4(1):4-16.
- Nichols RG, et al. Interplay Between the Host, the Human Microbiome, and Drug Metabolism. Hum Genomics. 2019 Jun;13(1):27.
- Nieman DC, Wentz LM. The compelling link between physical activity and the body's defense system. J Sport Heal Sci. 2019;8(3):201-17.
- Quagliani D, Felt-Gunderson P. Closing America's Fiber Intake Gap: Communication Strategies From a Food and Fiber Summit. Am J Lifestyle Med. 2017 Jul;11(1):80-5.
- Rodríguez JM, et al. The composition of the gut microbiota throughout life, with an emphasis on early life. Microb Ecol Heal Dis. 2015 Feb;26(0):26050.
- Rowland I, et al. Gut microbiota functions: metabolism of nutrients and other food components. Eur J Nutr. 2017/04/09. 2018 Feb;57(1):1-24.
- Sekirov I, et al. Gut microbiota in health and disease. Physiol Rev. 2010 Jul;90(3):859-904.
- Sender R, et al. Are We Really Vastly Outnumbered? Revisiting the Ratio of Bacterial to Host Cells in Humans. Cell. 2016;164(3):337-40.
- Slavin J. Fiber and prebiotics: Mechanisms and health benefits. Nutrients. 2013 Apr;5(4):1417-35.
- Tun HM, et al. Exposure to household furry pets influences the gut microbiota of infants at 3-4 months following various birth scenarios. Microbiome. 2017;5(1):40.
- Tuso PJ, et al. Nutritional update for physicians: plant-based diets. Perm J. 2013;17(2):61-6.
- Valdes AM, et al. Role of the gut microbiota in nutrition and health. BMJ. 2018 Jun;361:36-44.
- Yang CL, et al. Increased hunger, food cravings, food reward, and portion size selection after sleep curtailment in women without obesity. Nutrients. 2019 Mar;11(3):663.
- Zhang YJ, et al. Impacts of gut bacteria on human health and diseases. Int J Mol Sci. 2015 Apr;16(4):7493-519.

CHAPTER 8 – DIET NO-GO'S IN PANDEMIC TIMES

- Agócs R, et al. Is too much salt harmful? Yes. Pediatric Nephrology. 2019 Nov 28:1-9.
- Andersen CJ. Impact of dietary cholesterol on the pathophysiology of infectious and autoimmune disease. Nutrients. 2018 Jun;10(6):764.
- Antman EM, et al. Stakeholder discussion to reduce population-wide sodium intake and decrease sodium in the food supply: a conference report from the American Heart Association Sodium Conference 2013 Planning Group. Circulation. 2014 Jun 24;129(25):e660-79.
- Arackal BS, Benegal V. Prevalence of sexual dysfunction in male subjects with alcohol dependence. Indian Journal of Psychiatry. 2007 Apr;49(2):109.
- Attwood AS, Munafò MR. Effects of acute alcohol consumption and processing of emotion in faces: implications for understanding alcohol-related aggression. Journal of psychopharmacology. 2014 Aug;28(8):719-32.
- Badrick E, et al. The relationship between alcohol consumption and cortisol secretion in an aging cohort. The Journal of Clinical Endocrinology & Metabolism. 2008 Mar 1;93(3):750-7.
- Brooke-Taylor S, et al. Systematic review of the gastrointestinal effects of A1 compared with A2 -casein. Advances in nutrition. 2017 Sep;8(5):739-48.
- Brumback T, et al. Effects of alcohol on psychomotor performance and perceived impairment in heavy binge social drinkers. Drug and alcohol dependence. 2007 Nov 2;91(1):10-7.
- Calhoun VD, et al. Alcohol intoxication effects on visual perception: an fMRI study. Human brain mapping. 2004 Jan;21(1):15-26.
- Cook NR, et al. Sodium and health–concordance and controversy. bmj. 2020 Jun 26;369.
- Della Corte KW, et al. Effect of dietary sugar intake on biomarkers of subclinical inflammation: a systematic review and meta-analysis of intervention studies. Nutrients. 2018 May;10(5):606.
- DiNicolantonio JJ, Lucan SC. The wrong white crystals: not salt but sugar as aetiological in hypertension and cardiometabolic disease. Open heart. 2014 Nov 1;1(1):e000167.
- Djoussé L, et al. Consumption of fried foods and risk of heart failure in the physicians' health study. Journal of the American Heart Association. 2015 Apr 23;4(4):e001740.
- Elitsur Y, Luk GD. Beta-casomorphin (BCM) and human colonic lamina propria lymphocyte proliferation. Clinical & experimental immunology. 1991 Sep;85(3):493-7.
- Evcili G, et al. Early and long period follow-up results of low glycemic index diet for migraine prophylaxis. Agri. 2018 Jan 8;30(1):8-11.
- Frassetto L, et al. A. Acid balance, dietary acid load, and bone effects–a controversial subject. Nutrients. 2018 Apr;10(4):517.
- Fuhrman J. The hidden dangers of fast and processed food. American journal of lifestyle medicine. 2018 Sep;12(5):375-81.
- Grivennikov SI, et al. M. Immunity, inflammation, and cancer. Cell. 2010 Mar 19;140(6):883-99.
- Husain K, et al. Alcohol-induced hypertension: Mechanism and prevention. World journal of cardiology. 2014 May 26;6(5):245.
- Iadecola C. Sugar and Alzheimer's disease: a bittersweet truth. nature neuroscience. 2015 Apr;18(4):477-8.
- Jacques A, et al. The impact of sugar consumption on stress driven, emotional and addictive behaviors. Neuroscience & Biobehavioral Reviews. 2019 Aug 1;103:178-99.
- Jakobsen LS, et al. Probabilistic approach for assessing cancer risk due to benzo [a] pyrene in barbecued meat: Informing advice for population groups. PloS one. 2018 Nov 8;13(11):e0207032.
- Jensen T, et al. Fructose and sugar: A major mediator of non-alcoholic fatty liver disease. Journal of hepatology. 2018 May 1;68(5):1063-75.
- Jeyaraman MM, et al. Dairy product consumption and development of cancer: an overview of reviews. BMJ open. 2019 Jan 1;9(1):e023625.
- Jobin K, et al. A high-salt diet compromises antibacterial neutrophil responses through hormonal perturbation. Science translational medicine. 2020 Mar 25;12(536).
- Knowles J, et al. Iodine intake through processed food: case studies from Egypt, Indonesia, the Philippines, the Russian Federation and Ukraine, 2010–2015. Nutrients. 2017 Aug;9(8):797.
- Knüppel A, et al. Sugar intake from sweet food and beverages, common mental disorder and depression: prospective findings from the Whitehall II study. Scientific reports. 2017 Jul 27;7(1):1-0.
- Laugesen M, Elliott RB. Ischaemic heart disease, Type 1 diabetes, and cow milk A1 -casein.
- Lechner WV, et al. Effects of alcohol-induced working memory decline on alcohol consumption and adverse consequences of use. Psychopharmacology. 2016 Jan 1;233(1):83-8.
- Leggio L, et al. Blood glucose level, alcohol heavy drinking, and alcohol craving during treatment for alcohol dependence: results from the Combined Pharmacotherapies and Behavioral Interventions for Alcohol Dependence (COMBINE) Study. Alcoholism: Clinical and Experimental Research. 2009 Sep;33(9):1539-44.
- Leisegang K. Malnutrition and obesity. InOxidants, antioxidants and impact of the oxidative status in male reproduction 2019 Jan 1 (pp. 117-134). Academic Press.
- Mahtani KR. Simple advice to reduce salt intake. British Journal of General Practice. 2009 Oct 1;59(567):786-7.
- Makarem N, et al. Consumption of sugars, sugary foods, and sugary beverages in relation to adiposity-related cancer risk in the Framingham Offspring Cohort (1991–2013). Cancer Prevention Research. 2018 Jun 1;11(6):347-58.
- Mantantzis K, et al. Sugar rush or sugar crash? A meta-analysis of carbohydrate effects on mood. Neuroscience & Biobehavioral Reviews. 2019 Jun 1;101:45-67.
- Michalopoulos GK. Liver regeneration. Journal of cellular physiology. 2007 Nov;213(2):286-300.
- Miranda PM, et al. High salt diet exacerbates colitis in mice by decreasing Lactobacillus levels and butyrate production. Microbiome. 2018 Dec;6(1):1-7.
- Morgan MY. The prognosis and outcome of alcoholic liver disease. Alcohol and Alcoholism (Oxford, Oxfordshire). Supplement. 1994 Jan 1;2:335-43.
- Moynihan P. Sugars and dental caries: evidence for setting a recommended threshold for intake. Advances in nutrition. 2016 Jan;7(1):149-56.
- Mucci LA, Wilson KM. Acrylamide intake through diet and human cancer risk. Journal of agricultural and food chemistry. 2008 Aug 13;56(15):6013-9.
- Myles IA. Fast food fever: reviewing the impacts of the Western diet on immunity. Nutr J. 2014 Jun 17;13:61.
- Nguyen DD, et al. Formation and Degradation of Beta-casomorphins in Dairy Processing. Crit Rev Food Sci Nutr. 2015;55(14):1955-67.

- Osna N, et al. Alcoholic liver disease: pathogenesis and current management. Alcohol research: current reviews. 2017;38(2):147.
- Pinnock CB, et al. Relationship between milk intake and mucus production in adult volunteers challenged with rhinovirus-2. Am Rev Respir Dis. 1990 Feb 1;141(2):352-6.
- Price A, Stanhope KL. Understanding the Impact of Added Sugar Consumption on Risk for Type 2 Diabetes. Journal of the California Dental Association. 2016 Oct 1;44(10):619-26.
- Rippe JM, Angelopoulos TJ. Sugars, obesity, and cardiovascular disease: results from recent randomized control trials. European journal of nutrition. 2016 Nov;55(2):45-53.
- Santarelli RL, et al. Processed meat and colorectal cancer: a review of epidemiologic and experimental evidence. Nutrition and cancer. 2008 Mar 17;60(2):131-44.
- Sarkar D, et al. Alcohol and the immune system. Alcohol research: current reviews. 2015;37(2):153.
- Satokari R. High intake of sugar and the balance between pro-and anti-inflammatory gut bacteria.
- Schrieks IC, et al. The effect of alcohol consumption on insulin sensitivity and glycemic status: a systematic review and meta-analysis of intervention studies. Diabetes Care. 2015 Apr;38(4):723-32.
- Seitz HK, Becker P. Alcohol metabolism and cancer risk. Alcohol Research & Health. 2007;30(1):38.
- Sharma C, et al. Advanced glycation End-products (AGEs): an emerging concern for processed food industries. Journal of food science and technology. 2015 Dec;52(12):7561-76.
- Smith R, et al. A pilot study to determine the short-term effects of a low glycemic load diet on hormonal markers of acne: a nonrandomized, parallel, controlled feeding trial. Molecular nutrition & food research. 2008 Jun;52(6):718-26.
- Stanhope KL. Sugar consumption, metabolic disease and obesity: The state of the controversy. Critical reviews in clinical laboratory sciences. 2016 Jan 2;53(1):52-67.
- Statovci D, et al. The impact of western diet and nutrients on the microbiota and immune response at mucosal interfaces. Frontiers in immunology. 2017 Jul 28;8:838.
- Stein MD, Friedmann PD. Disturbed sleep and its relationship to alcohol use. Substance abuse. 2006 Feb 15;26(1):1-3.
- Tall AR, Yvan-Charvet L. Cholesterol, inflammation and innate immunity. Nat Rev Immunol. 2015 Feb;15(2):104-16.
- Tangvoranuntakul P, et al. Human uptake and incorporation of an immunogenic nonhuman dietary sialic acid. Proceedings of the National Academy of Sciences. 2003 Oct 14;100(21):12045-50.
- Uribarri J, et al. Advanced glycation end products in foods and a practical guide to their reduction in the diet. J Am Diet Assoc. 2010 Jun;110(6):911-16.e12.
- Wallace TC, et al. Current Sodium Intakes in the United States and the Modelling of Glutamate's Incorporation into Select Savory Products. Nutrients. 2019 Nov 7;11(11):2691.
- Westover AN, Marangell LB. A cross-national relationship between sugar consumption and major depression? Depress Anxiety. 2002;16(3):118-20.
- Yide Q, et al. Effect of# beta#-casomorphin-7 on growth, growth-related hormone and GHR mRNA expression in rats. [Ying Yang xue Bao] Acta Nutrimenta Sinica. 2004 Jan 1;26(2):112-5.
- Yu S, Zhang G, Jin LH. A high-sugar diet affects cellular and humoral immune responses in Drosophila. Experimental cell research. 2018 Jul 15;368(2):215-24.

CHAPTER 9 – DRESS TO SUPPRESS

- Aristizábal B, González Á. Innate immune system - Autoimmunity - NCBI Bookshelf [Internet]. El Rosario University Press. 2013. p. 31–47. Available from: https://www.ncbi.nlm.nih.gov/books/NBK459455/
- Bloomfield SF, et al. The infection risks associated with clothing and household linens in home and everyday life settings, and the role of laundry. International Scientific Forum on Home Hygiene. 2011.
- Bockmühl DP, et al. Laundry and textile hygiene in healthcare and beyond. Microb Cell. 2019 Jul 1;6(7):299-306.
- Callewaert C, et al. Bacterial Exchange in Household Washing Machines. Front Microbiol. 2015 Dec 8;6:1381.
- Castellani JW, Young AJ. Human physiological responses to cold exposure: Acute responses and acclimatization to prolonged exposure. Autonomic Neuroscience. 2016 Apr 1;196:63-74.
- Cohen RA. The Ongoing History of Harm Caused and Hidden by the Viscose Rayon and Cellophane Industry. Am J Public Health. 2018 Oct;108(10):1274-5.
- Crini G, et al. Applications of hemp in textiles, paper industry, insulation and building materials, horticulture, animal nutrition, food and beverages, nutraceuticals, cosmetics and hygiene, medicine, agrochemistry, energy production and environment: a review. Environ Chem Lett. 2020; 18: 1451–1476.
- De Sousa J, et al. The effects of a moisture-wicking fabric shirt on the physiological and perceptual responses during acute exercise in the heat. Vol. 45, Applied Ergonomics. 2014. p. 1447-53.
- Eriksson H, et al. Body temperature in general population samples. The study of men born in 1913 and 1923. Acta Med Scand. 1985;217(4):347-52.
- Eungpinichpong W, et al. Effects of restrictive clothing on lumbar range of motion and trunk muscle activity in young adult worker manual material handling. Appl Ergon. 2013 Nov;44(6):1024-32.
- Evans SS, et al. Fever and the thermal regulation of immunity: The immune system feels the heat. Vol. 15, Nature Reviews Immunology. 2015. p. 335-49.
- Fowler JF, et al. Effects of merino wool on atopic dermatitis using clinical, quality of life, and physiological outcome measures. Vol. 30, Dermatitis. 2019. p. 198-206.
- Galloway S. Dehydration, rehydration, and exercise in the heat: rehydration strategies for athletic competition. Canadian journal of applied physiology. 1999 Apr 1;24(2):188-200.
- Gambichler T, et al. Protection against ultraviolet radiation by commercial summer clothing: Need for standardised testing and labelling. Vol. 1, BMC Dermatology. 2001.
- Gass E, Gass G. Thermoregulatory responses to repeated warm water immersion in subjects who are paraplegic. Spinal Cord. 2001 Mar;39(3):149-55.
- Gerba C, Kennedy D. Enteric virus survival during household laundering and impact of disinfection with sodium hypochlorite. Appl Environ Microbiol. 2007 Jul;73(14):4425-8.
- Gralton J, et al. Personal clothing as a potential vector of respiratory virus transmission in childcare settings. J Med Virol. 2015 Jun;87(6):925-30.
- Grice EA, Segre JA. The skin microbiome. Vol. 9, Nature Reviews Microbiology. 2011. p. 244-53.
- Hadland D, et al. Heat and cold tolerance: relation to body weight. Postgrad Med. 1974 Apr;55(4):75-80.
- Hifumi T, et al. Heat stroke. J Intensive Care. 2018 May 22;6:30.
- Hu G, et al. Effect of cold stress on immunity in rats. Experimental and therapeutic medicine. 2016 Jan 1;11(1):33-42.
- Hung M, et al. Influence of silk clothing therapy in patients with atopic dermatitis. Dermatol Reports. 2019 Dec 22;11(2):8176.
- Jung S, et al. Influence of polyester spacer fabric, cotton, chloroprene rubber, and silicone on microclimatic and morphologic physiologic skin parameters in vivo. Skin Res Technol. 2019 May;25(3):389-398.
- Koop L, Tadi P. Physiology, Heat Loss. [Updated 2020 Jul 27]. In: StatPearls [Internet]. Treasure Island (FL): StatPearls Publishing; 2021 Jan-.
- Ladaresta F, et al. Chemicals from textiles to skin: an in vitro permeation study of benzothiazole. Vol. 25, Environmental Science and Pollution Research. 2018. p. 24629-38.
- Lee-Chiong Jr T, Stitt J. Disorders of temperature regulation. Comprehensive therapy. 1995 Dec 1;21(12):697-704.
- Léonard A, et al. Mutagenicity, carcinogenicity, and teratogenicity of acrylonitrile. Mutat Res. 1999 May;436(3):263-83.
- Miyatsuji A, et al. Effects of clothing pressure caused by different types of brassieres on autonomic nervous system activity evaluated by heart rate variability power spectral analysis. Journal of physiological anthropology and applied human science. 2002; 21: 67-74. 10.2114/jpa.21.67.
- Morais DS, et al. Antimicrobial approaches for textiles: From research to market. Vol. 9, Materials. 2016.
- Mu F, et al. Structural characterization and association of ovine Dickkopf-1 gene with wool production and quality traits in Chinese merino. Vol. 8, Genes. 2017.
- Nieman D, Wentz L. The compelling link between physical activity and the body's defense system. Journal of sport and health science. 2019 May 1;8(3):201-17.
- Nurul Fazita M, et al. Green Composites Made of Bamboo Fabric and Poly (Lactic) Acid for Packaging Applications-A Review. Materials (Basel). 2016 Jun 1;9(6):435.
- Osilla E, et al. Physiology, Temperature Regulation. [Updated 2021 May 7]. In: StatPearls [Internet]. Treasure Island (FL): StatPearls Publishing; 2021 Jan-.
- Rovira J, et al. Human exposure to trace elements through the skin by direct contact with clothing: Risk assessment. Vol. 140, Environmental Research. 2015. p. 308-16.
- Shephard R, Shek P. Cold exposure and immune function. Canadian journal of physiology and pharmacology. 1998 Sep 1;76(9):828-36.
- Shin M, et al. The effects of fabric for sleepwear and bedding on sleep at ambient temperatures of 17°C and 22°C. Vol. 8, Nature and Science of Sleep. 2016. p. 121-31.
- Sone Y, et al. Effects of skin pressure by clothing on digestion and orocecal transit time of food. Journal of Physiological anthropology and applied human science. 2000 May 30;19(3):157-63.
- Starkie R, et al. Heat stress, cytokines, and the immune response to exercise. Brain Behav Immun. 2005 Sep;19(5):404-12.
- Suran M. A planet too rich in fibre: Microfibre pollution may have major consequences on the environment and human health. EMBO Rep. 2018 Sep;19(9):e46701.
- Svedman C, et al. Textile Contact Dermatitis: How Fabrics Can Induce Dermatitis. Curr Treat Options Allergy. 2019; 6:103-111 (2019).
- Takasu N, et al. The effects of skin pressure by clothing on whole gut transit time and amount of feces. J Physiol Anthropol Appl Human Sci. 2000 May;19(3):151-6.
- Yoo W. Effect of wearing tight pants on the trunk flexion and pelvic tilting angles in the stand-to-sit movement and a seated posture. J Phys Ther Sci. 2016 Jan;28(1):93-5.
- Yueping W, et al. Structures of bamboo fiber for textiles. Text. Res. J. 2010;80:334-343.

CHAPTER 10 – ADOPT A CHINCHILLA! NOT

- Abebe E, et al. Review on major food-borne zoonotic bacterial pathogens. Journal of Tropical Medicine. 2020 Jun 29;2020.
- Anderson NL. Pet rodents. Saunders Manual of Small Animal Practice. 2006:1881.
- Bedford J, et al. A new twenty-first century science for effective epidemic response. Nature. 2019 Nov;575(7781):130-6.
- Bergen-Cico D, et al. Dog ownership and training reduces post-traumatic stress symptoms and increases self-compassion among veterans: results of a longitudinal control Study. The Journal of Alternative and Complementary Medicine. 2018 Dec 1;24(12):1166-75.
- Bir C, et al. Familiarity and use of veterinary services by US resident dog and cat owners. Vol. 10, Animals. 2020.
- Bjelland AM, et al. Prevalence of Salmonella serovars isolated from reptiles in Norwegian zoos. Acta Veterinaria Scandinavica. 2020 Dec;62(1):1-9.
- Cherry JD. The chronology of the 2002-2003 SARS mini pandemic. Paediatric respiratory reviews. 2004 Dec 1;5(4):262-9.
- Chomel BB, et al. Wildlife, exotic pets, and emerging zoonoses. Emerging infectious diseases. 2007 Jan;13(1):6.
- Chomel BB. Zoonoses. Encyclopedia of Microbiology. 2009:820.
- Christian H, et al. Understanding the relationship between dog ownership and children's physical activity and sedentary behaviour. Pediatric Obesity. 2013 Oct;8(5):392-403.
- Clayton LA, McDermott C. Fish Behavior for the Exotic Pet Practitioner. The Veterinary Clinics of North America. Exotic Animal Practice. 2021 Jan;24(1):211-27.
- Cohen FS. How viruses invade cells. Biophysical journal. 2016 Mar 8;110(5):1028-32.
- Control C for D. Farm Animals | Healthy Pets, Healthy People | CDC [Internet]. 2020. Available from: https://www.cdc.gov/healthypets/pets/farm-animals.html
- Cottam EM, et al. Full sequencing of viral genomes: practical strategies used for the amplification and characterization of foot-and-mouth disease virus. InMolecular Epidemiology of Microorganisms 2009 (pp. 217-230). Humana Press, Totowa, NJ.
- Croft DR, et al. Occupational risks during a monkeypox outbreak, Wisconsin, 2003. Emerging infectious diseases. 2007 Aug;13(8):1150.
- Esch KJ, Petersen CA. Transmission and epidemiology of zoonotic protozoal diseases of companion animals. Clinical microbiology reviews. 2013 Jan;26(1):58.
- Facts P. Pet Population and Ownership Trends in the U . S . 2017. Does the US Have a Population Problem?
- Failloux AB, Moutailler S. Zoonotic aspects of vector-borne infections. Rev Sci Technol. 2015 Apr 1;34(1):175-83.
- Ferrell ST. Amphibian Behavior for the Exotic Pet Practitioner. Veterinary Clinics: Exotic Animal Practice. 2021 Jan;24(1):197-210.
- Gleeson M, Petritz OA. Emerging Infectious Diseases of Rabbits. Veterinary Clinics: Exotic Animal Practice. 2020 May 1;23(2):249-61.
- Harris LM. Ferret wellness management and environmental enrichment. The veterinary clinics of North America. Exotic animal practice. 2015 May;18(2):233.
- Hawkins RD, Williams JM. Childhood attachment to pets: Associations between pet attachment, attitudes to animals, compassion, and humane behaviour. International journal of environmental research and public health. 2017 May;14(5):490.
- Hess L. The changing face of bird and exotic pet practice. Journal of avian medicine and surgery. 2013 Dec;27(4):315-8.
- Hilliard J. Monkey B virus. Human herpesviruses: biology, therapy, and immunoprophylaxis. 2007.
- Hutchison ML, et al. The air-borne distribution of zoonotic agents from livestock waste spreading and microbiological risk to fresh produce from contaminated irrigation sources. J Appl Microbiol. 2008 Sep;105(3):848-57.
- Jennings LB. Potential benefits of pet ownership in health promotion. Journal of Holistic Nursing. 1997 Dec;15(4):358-72.
- Karatepe M. Struggle against typhus in the Caucasian front during the 1st World War. Yeni tip tarihi arastirmalari= The new history of medicine studies. 2002 Jan 1;8:107-62.
- Karlinsky A, Kobak D. The World Mortality Dataset: Tracking excess mortality across countries during the COVID-19 pandemic. medRxiv. 2021 Jan 1.
- Lai S, et al. Global epidemiology of avian influenza A H5N1 virus infection in humans, 1997–2015: a systematic review of individual case data. The Lancet Infectious Diseases. 2016 Jul 1;16(7):e108-18.
- Leligdowicz A, et al. Ebola virus disease and critical illness. Critical Care. 2016 Dec;20(1):1-4.
- Ligon BL. Monkeypox: a review of the history and emergence in the Western hemisphere. InSeminars in pediatric infectious diseases 2004 Oct 1 (Vol. 15, No. 4, pp. 280-287). WB Saunders.
- Lin CN. Impacts on human health caused by zoonoses. Biological toxins and bioterrorism. 2015;1:211.
- Mahalingam S, et al. Hendra virus: an emerging paramyxovirus in Australia. The Lancet infectious diseases. 2012 Oct 1;12(10):799-807.
- Marshall-Pescini S, et al. The role of oxytocin in the dog–owner relationship. Animals. 2019 Oct;9(10):792.
- Martini M, et al. The Spanish Influenza Pandemic: a lesson from history 100 years after 1918. Journal of preventive medicine and hygiene. 2019 Mar;60(1):E64.
- Mendoza-Roldan J, et al. Zoonotic parasites of reptiles: a crawling threat. Trends in parasitology. 2020 May 7.
- Mobaraki K, Ahmadzadeh J. Current epidemiological status of Middle East respiratory syndrome coronavirus in the world from 1.1. 2017 to 17.1. 2018: a cross-sectional study. BMC infectious diseases. 2019 Dec;19(1):1-5.
- Overgaauw PAM, et al. One health perspective on the human-companion animal relationship with emphasis on zoonotic aspects. Vol. 17, International Journal of Environmental Research and Public Health. 2020.
- Petersson M, et al. Oxytocin and cortisol levels in dog owners and their dogs are associated with behavioral patterns: An exploratory study. Frontiers in psychology. 2017 Oct 13;8:1796.
- Polheber JP, Matchock RL. The presence of a dog attenuates cortisol and heart rate in the Trier Social Stress Test compared to human friends. Journal of behavioral medicine. 2014 Oct;37(5):860-7.
- Powell L, et al. Expectations for dog ownership: Perceived physical, mental and psychosocial health consequences among prospective adopters. PLoS One. 2018 Jul 6;13(7):e0200276.
- Qureshi AI, et al. Cat ownership and the Risk of Fatal Cardiovascular Diseases. Results from the Second National Health and Nutrition Examination Study Mortality Follow-up Study. Journal of vascular and interventional neurology. 2009 Jan;2(1):132.
- Raikova SV, Zav'ialov AI. Typhus fever morbidity among the military personnel and civilians in the regions around Volga river during World War I. Voenno-meditsinskii zhurnal. 2013 Jul 1;334(7):56-61.
- Rodrigo-Claverol M, et al. Animal-Assisted Therapy Improves Communication and Mobility among Institutionalized People with Cognitive Impairment. International journal of environmental research and public health. 2020 Jan;17(16):5899.
- Salyer SJ, et al. Prioritizing zoonoses for global health capacity building—themes from One Health zoonotic disease workshops in 7 countries, 2014–2016. Emerging infectious diseases. 2017 Dec;23(Suppl 1):S55.
- Sanjuán R, Domingo-Calap P. Mechanisms of viral mutation. Cellular and molecular life sciences. 2016 Dec;73(23):4433-48.
- Saunders-Hastings PR, Krewski D. Reviewing the history of pandemic influenza: understanding patterns of emergence and transmission. Pathogens. 2016 Dec;5(4):66.
- Shader RI. Zoonotic viruses: the mysterious leap from animals to man. Clinical therapeutics. 2018 Aug;40(8):1225.
- Shariff M. Nipah virus infection: a review. Epidemiology & Infection. 2019;147.
- Simonsen L, et al. Global mortality estimates for the 2009 Influenza Pandemic from the GLaMOR project: a modeling study. PLoS Med. 2013 Nov 26;10(11):e1001558.
- Simpson A. Effect of household pet ownership on infant immune response and subsequent sensitization. Journal of asthma and allergy. 2010;3:131.
- Souza MJ. One health: zoonoses in the exotic animal practice. Veterinary Clinics: Exotic Animal Practice. 2011 Sep 1;14(3):421-6.
- Strathdee SA, et al. What the HIV pandemic experience can teach the United States about the COVID-19 response. Journal of acquired immune deficiency syndromes (1999). 2021 Jan 1;86(1):1.
- Taubenberger JK. The origin and virulence of the 1918 "Spanish" influenza virus. Proceedings of the American Philosophical Society. 2006 Mar;150(1):86.
- Vergles Rataj A, et al. Parasites in pet reptiles. Acta veterinaria scandinavica. 2011;53(33):1-20.
- Villarreal LP. Evolution of viruses. Encyclopedia of Virology. 2008:174.
- Whiley H, et al. A review of Salmonella and squamates (lizards, snakes and amphisbians): implications for public health. Pathogens. 2017 Sep;6(3):38.

CHAPTER 11 – EAT, DRINK, & BE STRONG

- Åkerström S, et al. Nitric oxide inhibits the replication cycle of severe acute respiratory syndrome coronavirus. Journal of virology. 2005 Feb;79(3):1966.
- Arshad MS, et al. Coronavirus disease (COVID-19) and immunity booster green foods: A mini review. Food Science & Nutrition. 2020 Aug;8(8):3971-6.
- Asemani Y, et al. Allium vegetables for possible future of cancer treatment. Phytotherapy Research. 2019 Dec;33(12):3019-39.
- Bahrami A, et al. A. Legume intake and risk of nonalcoholic fatty liver disease. Indian Journal of Gastroenterology. 2019 Feb;38(1):55-60.
- Bazzano LA, et al. Legume consumption and risk of coronary heart disease in US men and women: NHANES I Epidemiologic Follow-up Study. Arch Intern Med. 2001;161(21):2573-2578.
- Bazzano LA, et al. Non-soy legume consumption lowers cholesterol levels: a meta-analysis of randomized controlled trials. Nutrition, metabolism and cardiovascular diseases. 2011 Feb 1;21(2):94-103.
- Bendich A. Physiological role of antioxidants in the immune system. Journal of Dairy Science. 1993 Sep 1;76(9):2789-94.
- Borek C. Dietary antioxidants and human cancer. Integrative cancer therapies. 2004 Dec;3(4):333-41.
- Castro-Acosta ML, et al. Berries and anthocyanins: promising functional food ingredients with postprandial glycaemia-lowering effects. Proceedings of the Nutrition Society. 2016 Aug;75(3):342-55.
- Cernava T, et al. Enterobacteriaceae dominate the core microbiome and contribute to the resistome of arugula (Eruca sativa Mill.). Microbiome. 2019 Dec;7(1):1-2.
- Coleman JW. Nitric oxide in immunity and inflammation. International immunopharmacology. 2001 Aug 1;1(8):1397-406.
- Forman HJ, Zhang H, Rinna A. Glutathione: overview of its protective roles, measurement, and biosynthesis. Molecular aspects of medicine. 2009 Feb 1;30(1-2):1-2.
- Fukagawa NK, et al. High-carbohydrate, high-fiber diets increase peripheral insulin sensitivity in healthy young and old adults. The American journal of clinical nutrition. 1990 Sep 1;52(3):524-8.
- Gamba M, et al. Bioactive compounds and nutritional composition of Swiss chard (Beta vulgaris L. var. cicla and flavescens): a systematic review. Critical reviews in food science and nutrition. 2020 Aug 6:1-6.

REFERENCES

- Guo S, et al. A review of phytochemistry, metabolite changes, and medicinal uses of the common sunflower seed and sprouts (Helianthus annuus L.). Chemistry Central Journal. 2017 Dec;11(1):1-0.
- Hemilä H. Vitamin C and infections. Nutrients. 2017 Apr;9(4):339.
- Jayachandran M, et al. A critical review on health promoting benefits of edible mushrooms through gut microbiota. International journal of molecular sciences. 2017 Sep;18(9):1934.
- Kajla P, et al. Flaxseed—a potential functional food source. Journal of food science and technology. 2015 Apr;52(4):1857-71.
- Kapusta-Duch J, et al. The beneficial effects of Brassica vegetables on human health. Roczniki Państwowego Zakładu Higieny. 2012;63(4).
- Karaś M, et al. Antioxidant activity of protein hydrolysates from raw and heat-treated yellow string beans (Phaseolus vulgaris L.). Acta Scientiarum Polonorum Technologia Alimentaria. 2014 Dec 30;13(4).
- Kim JK, et al. Comparative analysis of glucosinolates and metabolite profiling of green and red mustard (brassica juncea) hairy roots. 3 Biotech. 2018 Sep;8(9):1-0.
- Kothari D, et al. Allium Flavonols: Health Benefits, Molecular Targets, and Bioavailability. Antioxidants. 2020 Sep;9(9):888.
- Lanza E, et al. High dry bean intake and reduced risk of advanced colorectal adenoma recurrence among participants in the polyp prevention trial. The Journal of nutrition. 2006 Jul 1;136(7):1896-903.
- Leizer C, et al. The composition of hemp seed oil and its potential as an important source of nutrition. Journal of Nutraceuticals, functional & medical foods. 2000 Dec 1;2(4):35-53.
- Li Y, et al. Quercetin, Inflammation and Immunity. Nutrients. 2016;8(3):167. Published 2016 Mar 15. doi:10.3390/nu8030167
- Lovejoy JC. The influence of dietary fat on insulin resistance. Current diabetes reports. 2002 Oct 1;2(5):435-40.
- Luiking YC, et al. Regulation of nitric oxide production in health and disease. Current opinion in clinical nutrition and metabolic care. 2010 Jan;13(1):97.
- Messina V. Nutritional and health benefits of dried beans. The American journal of clinical nutrition. 2014 Jul 1;100(suppl_1):437S-42S.
- Michel JB. Rôle du monoxyde d'azote endothélial dans la régulation de la vasomotricité [Role of endothelial nitric oxide in the regulation of the vasomotor system]. Pathol Biol (Paris). 1998;46(3):181-189.
- Milkowski A, et al. Nutritional epidemiology in the context of nitric oxide biology: A risk-benefit evaluation for dietary nitrite and nitrate. Nitric oxide. 2010 Feb 15;22(2):110-9.
- Mirvish SS. Role of N-nitroso compounds (NOC) and N-nitrosation in etiology of gastric, esophageal, nasopharyngeal and bladder cancer and contribution to cancer of known exposures to NOC. Cancer letters. 1995 Jun 29;93(1):17-48.
- Monk JM, et al. Navy and black bean supplementation primes the colonic mucosal microenvironment to improve gut health. The Journal of nutritional biochemistry. 2017 Nov 1;49:89-100.
- Moreno-Ortega A, et al. Changes in the antioxidant activity and metabolite profile of three onion varieties during the elaboration of 'black onion'. Food chemistry. 2020 May 1;311:125958.
- Moser MA, Chun OK. Vitamin C and heart health: a review based on findings from epidemiologic studies. International journal of molecular sciences. 2016 Aug;17(8):1328.
- Mzoughi Z, et al. Wild edible Swiss chard leaves (Beta vulgaris L. var. cicla): Nutritional, phytochemical composition and biological activities. Food Research International. 2019 May 1;119:612-21.
- Pathak N, et al. Value addition in sesame: A perspective on bioactive components for enhancing utility and profitability. Pharmacognosy reviews. 2014 Jul;8(16):147.
- Robbins RA, Grisham MB. Nitric oxide. The international journal of biochemistry & cell biology. 1997 Jun 1;29(6):857-60.
- Roberts JL, Moreau R. Functional properties of spinach (Spinacia oleracea L.) phytochemicals and bioactives. Food & function. 2016;7(8):3337-53.
- Šamec D, et al. Kale (Brassica oleracea var. acephala) as a superfood: Review of the scientific evidence behind the statement. Critical reviews in food science and nutrition. 2019 Aug 22;59(15):2411-22.
- Sathe SK. Dry bean protein functionality. Critical reviews in biotechnology. 2002 Jan 1;22(2):175-223.
- Suleria HA, et al. Onion: Nature protection against physiological threats. Critical reviews in food science and nutrition. 2015 Jan 2;55(1):50-66.
- Sverdlov AL, et al. Aging of the nitric oxide system: are we as old as our NO?. Journal of the American Heart Association. 2014 Aug 18;3(4):e000973.
- Thompson SV, et al. Bean and rice meals reduce postprandial glycemic response in adults with type 2 diabetes: a cross-over study. Nutrition Journal. 2012 Dec;11(1):1-7.
- Turner TF, et al. Dietary adherence and satisfaction with a bean-based high-fiber weight loss diet: a pilot study. International Scholarly Research Notices. 2013.
- Vega-Galvez A, et al. Antioxidant, functional properties and health-promoting potential of native South American berries: a review. Journal of the Science of Food and Agriculture. 2021 Jan 30;101(2):364-78.
- Villarreal-Calderón JR, et al. Interplay between the Adaptive Immune System and Insulin Resistance in Weight Loss Induced by Bariatric Surgery. Oxid Med Cell Longev. 2019;2019:3940739. Published 2019 Dec 6.
- Wu G, Meininger CJ. Regulation of nitric oxide synthesis by dietary factors. Annu Rev Nutr. 2002;22:61-86.
- Yu S, et al. A high-sugar diet affects cellular and humoral immune responses in Drosophila. Vol. 368, Experimental Cell Research. 2018. p. 215-24.
- Zhang JJ, et al. Bioactivities and health benefits of mushrooms mainly from China. Molecules. 2016 Jul;21(7):938.

CHAPTER 12 – LET THE SUN SHINE IN

- Alkozei A, et al. Exposure to blue light increases subsequent functional activation of the prefrontal cortex during performance of a working memory task. Sleep. 2016 Sep 1;39(9):1671-80.
- Allgrove J. Physiology of Calcium, Phosphate, Magnesium and Vitamin D. Endocr Dev. 2015;28:7-32.
- Aranow C. Vitamin D and the immune system. In: Journal of Investigative Medicine. BMJ Publishing Group; 2011. p. 881-6.
- Ash C, et al. Effect of wavelength and beam width on penetration in light-tissue interaction using computational methods. Lasers Med Sci. 2017 Nov;32(8):1909-18.
- Avci P, et al. Low-level laser (light) therapy (LLLT) in skin: Stimulating, healing, restoring. Semin Cutan Med Surg. 2013 Mar;32(1):41-52.
- Bae M, Kim H. Mini-Review on the Roles of Vitamin C, Vitamin D, and Selenium in the Immune System against COVID-19. Vol. 25, Molecules (Basel, Switzerland). NLM (Medline); 2020.
- Bonilla C, et al. Skin pigmentation, sun exposure and vitamin D levels in children of the avon longitudinal study of parents and children. BMC Public Health. 2014 Jun;14(1):1-10.
- Cardwell G, et al. A review of mushrooms as a potential source of dietary vitamin D. Vol. 10, Nutrients. MDPI AG; 2018.
- Cela EM, et al. Immune System Modulation Produced by Ultraviolet Radiation. In: Immunoregulatory Aspects of Immunotherapy. InTech; 2018.
- Chandra P, et al. Treatment of vitamin D deficiency with UV light in patients with malabsorption syndromes: A case series. Photodermatol Photoimmunol Photomed. 2007 Oct;23(5):179-85.
- Chaves ME, et al. Effects of low-power light therapy on wound healing: LASER x LED. Vol. 89, Anais Brasileiros de Dermatologia. Sociedade Brasileira de Dermatologia; 2014. p. 616-23.
- D'Orazio J, et al. UV radiation and the skin. Vol. 14, International Journal of Molecular Sciences. MDPI AG; 2013. p. 12222-48.
- Driller MW, et al. Hunger hormone and sleep responses to the built-in blue-light filter on an electronic device: A pilot study. In: Sleep Science. Brazilian Association of Sleep and Latin American Federation of Sleep Societies; 2019. p. 171-7.
- Eslami H, Jalili M. The role of environmental factors to transmission of SARS-CoV-2 (COVID-19). Vol. 10, AMB Express. Springer; 2020.
- Fahimipour AK, et al. Daylight exposure modulates bacterial communities associated with household dust 06 Biological Sciences 0605 Microbiology. Microbiome. 2018 Oct;6(1):1-13.
- Favero G, et al. Melatonin as an Anti-Inflammatory Agent Modulating Inflammasome Activation. Vol. 2017, International Journal of Endocrinology. Hindawi Limited; 2017.
- Forrest KYZ, Stuhldreher WL. Prevalence and correlates of vitamin D deficiency in US adults. Nutr Res. 2011 Jan;31(1):48-54.
- Garcia-Saenz A, et al. Evaluating the association between artificial light-at-night exposure and breast and prostate cancer risk in Spain (Mcc-spain study). Environ Health Perspect. 2018 Apr;126(4).
- Gwynne PJ, Gallagher MP. Light as a broad-spectrum antimicrobial. Front Microbiol. 2018 Feb;9(FEB).
- Hamblin MR. Mechanisms and applications of the anti-inflammatory effects of photobiomodulation. Vol. 4, AIMS Biophysics. American Institute of Mathematical Sciences; 2017. p. 337-61.
- Hernández JL, et al. Vitamin D Status in Hospitalized Patients with SARS-CoV-2 Infection. J Clin Endocrinol Metab. 2021 Mar;106(3):E1343-53.
- Holick MF. Evidence-based D-bate on health benefits of vitamin D revisited. Dermatoendocrinol. 2012 Apr;4(2):183-90.
- Hu D, et al. Red LED photobiomodulation reduces pain hypersensitivity and improves sensorimotor function following mild T10 hemicontusion spinal cord injury. J Neuroinflammation. 2016 Aug;13(1):1-15.
- Ibrahim MM, et al. Long-lasting antinociceptive effects of green light in acute and chronic pain in rats. Pain. 2017 Feb;158(2):347-60.
- Jniene A, et al. Perception of Sleep Disturbances due to Bedtime Use of Blue Light-Emitting Devices and Its Impact on Habits and Sleep Quality among Young Medical Students. Biomed Res Int. 2019;2019.
- Juzeniene A, Moan J. Beneficial effects of UV radiation other than via vitamin D production. Vol. 4, Dermato-Endocrinology. Taylor & Francis; 2012. p. 109-17.
- Keszler A, et al. Red/near infrared light stimulates release of an endothelium dependent vasodilator and rescues vascular dysfunction in a diabetes model. Free Radic Biol Med. 2017 Dec;113:157-64.
- Kimberly B, James R. P. Amber lenses to block blue light and improve sleep: A randomized trial. Chronobiol Int. 2009 Dec;26(8):1602-12.
- Knoop M, et al. Daylight: What makes the difference? Light Res Technol. 2020 May;52(3):423-42.
- Lee H, et al. Effects of exercise with or without light exposure on sleep quality and hormone reponses. J Exerc Nutr Biochem. 2014 Sep;18(3):293-9.
- Littlejohns TJ, et al. Vitamin D and the risk of dementia and Alzheimer disease. Neurology. 2014 Sep;83(10):920-8.
- MacDonald HM. Contributions of sunlight and diet to vitamin D status. Calcif Tissue Int. 2013 Feb;92(2):163-76.
- Martin LF, et al. Evaluation of green light exposure on headache frequency and quality of life in migraine patients: A preliminary one-way cross-over clinical trial. Cephalalgia. 2021 Feb;41(2):135-47.
- Mayerhöfer TG, Popp J. The electric field standing wave effect in infrared transflection spectroscopy. Spectrochim Acta - Part A Mol Biomol Spectrosc. 2018;191:283-9.
- Mead MN. Benefits of sunlight: a bright spot for human health. Vol. 116, Environmental health perspectives. National Institute of Environmental Health Sciences; 2008. p. A160.
- Minguillon J, et al. Blue lighting accelerates post-stress relaxation: Results of a preliminary study. PLoS One. 2017 Oct;12(10).
- Nair R, Maseeh A. Vitamin D: The sunshine vitamin. Vol. 3, Journal of Pharmacology and Pharmacotherapeutics. Wolters Kluwer -- Medknow Publications; 2012. p. 118-26.
- Nimitphong H, Holick MF. Vitamin D status and sun exposure in Southeast Asia. Dermatoendocrinol. 2013 Jan;5(1):34-7.
- Norman PE, Powell JT. Vitamin D and cardiovascular disease. Vol. 114, Circulation Research. Lippincott Williams and Wilkins; 2014. p. 379-93.
- Parva NR, et al. Prevalence of Vitamin D Deficiency and Associated Risk Factors in the US Population (2011-2012). Cureus. 2018 Jun;10(6).
- Phan TX, et al. Intrinsic photosensitivity enhances motility of T lymphocytes. Sci Rep. 2016 Dec;6(1):1-11.
- Plitnick B, et al. The effects of red and blue light on alertness and mood at night. Light Res Technol. 2010 Dec;42(4):449-58.
- Pugach IZ, Pugach S. Strong correlation between prevalence of severe vitamin D deficiency and population mortality rate from COVID-19 in Europe. Wien Klin Wochenschr. 2021 Apr;133(7-8):403-5.
- Shang YM, et al. White light-emitting diodes (LEDs) at domestic lighting levels and retinal injury in a rat model. Environ Health Perspect. 2014 Dec;122(3):269-76.
- Shen J, Tower J. Effects of light on aging and longevity. Vol. 53, Ageing Research Reviews. Elsevier Ireland Ltd; 2019. p. 100913.
- Szczepanik M. Melatonin and its influence on immune system. Vol. 58, Journal of Physiology and Pharmacology. 2007.
- Tafur J, Mills PJ. Low-intensity light therapy: Exploring the role of redox mechanisms. Vol. 26, Photomedicine and Laser Surgery. Mary Ann Liebert, Inc.; 2008. p. 323-8.
- Tähkämö L, et al. Systematic review of light exposure impact on human circadian rhythm. Vol. 36, Chronobiology International. Taylor and Francis Ltd; 2019. p. 151-70.
- Tarocco A, et al. Melatonin as a master regulator of cell death and inflammation: molecular mechanisms and clinical implications for newborn care. Vol. 10, Cell Death and Disease. Nature Publishing Group; 2019. p. 1-12.
- Tripkovic L, et al. Comparison of vitamin D2and vitamin D3 supplementation in raising serum 25-hydroxyvitamin D status: A systematic review and meta-analysis. Vol. 95, American Journal of Clinical Nutrition. American Society for Nutrition; 2012. p. 1357-64.
- Uccula A, et al. Colors, colored overlays, and reading skills. Vol. 5, Frontiers in Psychology. Frontiers Research Foundation; 2014.
- Wacker M, Holick MF. Sunlight and Vitamin D: A global perspective for health. Vol. 5, Dermato-Endocrinology. Landes Bioscience; 2013. p. 51-108.
- Wang Y, et al. Antimicrobial blue light inactivation of pathogenic microbes: State of the art. Drug Resist Updat. 2017 Nov;33-35:1-22.
- Wunsch A, Matuschka K. A controlled trial to determine the efficacy of red and near-infrared light treatment in patient satisfaction, reduction of fine lines, wrinkles, skin roughness, and intradermal collagen density increase. Photomed Laser Surg. 2014 Feb;32(2):93-100.
- Zhang R, Naughton DP. Vitamin D in health and disease: Current perspectives. Vol. 9, Nutrition Journal. BioMed Central; 2010. p. 1-13.
- Zhao ZC, et al. Research progress about the effect and prevention of blue light on eyes. Vol. 11, International Journal of Ophthalmology. International Journal of Ophthalmology (c/o Editorial Office); 2018. p. 1999-2003.
- Zielinska-Dabkowska KM, et al. LED light sources and their complex set-up for visually and biologically effective illumination for ornamental indoor plants. Sustain. 2019;11(9).

CHAPTER 13 – MOVE MORE, SIT LESS

- Bird SR, Hawley JA. Update on the effects of physical activity on insulin sensitivity in humans. BMJ open Sport Exerc Med. 2017 Mar;2(1):e000143-e000143.
- Blackstone EA, et al. The health and economic effects of counterfeit drugs. Am Heal drug benefits. 2014 Jun;7(4):216-24.
- Booth FW, et al. Lack of exercise is a major cause of chronic diseases. Compr Physiol. 2012 Apr;2(2):1143-211.
- Chau JY, et al. Daily sitting time and all-cause mortality: a meta-analysis. PLoS One. 2013 Nov;8(11):e80000-e80000.
- Church TS, et al. Trends over 5 decades in U.S. occupation-related physical activity and their associations with obesity. PLoS One. 2011/05/25. 2011;6(5):e19657-e19657.
- Daneshmandi H, et al. Adverse Effects of Prolonged Sitting Behavior on the General Health of Office Workers. J lifestyle Med. 2017/07/31. 2017 Jul;7(2):69-75.
- Dewitt S, et al. Office workers' experiences of attempts to reduce sitting-time: an exploratory, mixed-methods uncontrolled intervention pilot study. BMC Public Health. 2019;19(1):819.
- Dolezal BA, et al. Interrelationship between Sleep and Exercise: A Systematic Review. Adv Prev Med. 2017/03/26. 2017;2017:1364387.
- Ekelund U, et al. Does physical activity attenuate, or even eliminate, the detrimental association of sitting time with mortality? A harmonised meta-analysis of data from more than 1 million men and women. Lancet. 2016;388(10051):1302-10.
- El-Zayat SR, et al. Physiological process of fat loss. Bull Natl Res Cent. 2019;43(1):208.
- Fletcher GF, et al. Exercise Standards for Testing and Training. Circulation. 2001 Oct;104(14):1694-740.
- Galloza J, et al. Benefits of Exercise in the Older Population. Phys Med Rehabil Clin N Am. 2017;28(4):659-69.
- Hackney AC, Koltun KJ. The immune system and overtraining in athletes: clinical implications. Acta Clin Croat. 2012 Dec;51(4):633-41.
- Hadgraft NT, et al. Office workers' objectively assessed total and prolonged sitting time: Individual-level correlates and worksite variations. Prev Med Reports. 2016;4:184-91.
- Hamilton MT, et al. Too Little Exercise and Too Much Sitting: Inactivity Physiology and the Need for New Recommendations on Sedentary Behavior. Curr Cardiovasc Risk Rep. 2008 Jul;2(4):292-8.
- King AC, King DK. Physical activity for an aging population. Public Health Rev. 2010;32(2):401-26.
- Kohn LT, et al. Rapporteur's Report Session I: Origin of the problem: Malcolm Ross. Vol. 52, Regulatory Toxicology and Pharmacology. 2008.
- Kushner AM, et al. The Back Squat Part 2: Targeted Training Techniques to Correct Functional Deficits and Technical Factors that Limit Performance. Strength Cond J. 2015 Apr;37(2):13-60.
- Lai AT, et al. Climate change and human health. J Intern Med Taiwan. 2012;23(5):343-50.
- Lavie CJ, et al. Sedentary Behavior, Exercise, and Cardiovascular Health. Circ Res. 2019 Mar;124(5):799-815.
- Lee I-M, et al. Effect of physical inactivity on major non-communicable diseases worldwide: an analysis of burden of disease and life expectancy. Lancet (London, England). 2012 Jul;380(9838):219-29.
- Ma P, et al. Daily sedentary time and its association with risk for colorectal cancer in adults: A dose-response meta-analysis of prospective cohort studies. Medicine (Baltimore). 2017 Jun;96(22):e7049-e7049.
- Makki K, et al. Adipose tissue in obesity-related inflammation and insulin resistance: cells, cytokines, and chemokines. ISRN Inflamm. 2013 Dec;2013:139239.
- McFee RB. Nosocomial or hospital-acquired infections: an overview. Dis Mon. 2009 Jul;55(7):422-38.
- Myer GD, et al. The back squat: A proposed assessment of functional deficits and technical factors that limit performance. Strength Cond J. 2014 Dec;36(6):4-27.
- Owen N, et al. Too much sitting: the population health science of sedentary behavior. Exerc Sport Sci Rev. 2010 Jul;38(3):105-13.
- Reyes AZ, et al. Anti-inflammatory therapy for COVID-19 infection: the case for colchicine. Ann Rheum Dis. 2021 May;80(5):550 LP - 557.
- Thomas D, Apovian C. Macrophage functions in lean and obese adipose tissue. Metabolism. 2017/04/18. 2017 Jul;72:120-43.
- Thompson PD, et al. Exercise and Acute Cardiovascular Events. Circulation. 2007 May;115(17):2358-68.
- Thompson PD. Exercise Prescription and Proscription for Patients With Coronary Artery Disease. Circulation. 2005 Oct;112(15):2354-63.
- Tian D, Meng J. Exercise for Prevention and Relief of Cardiovascular Disease: Prognoses, Mechanisms, and Approaches. Oxid Med Cell Longev. 2019 Apr;2019:3756750.
- Vena D, et al. The Effect of Electrical Stimulation of the Calf Muscle on Leg Fluid Accumulation over a Long Period of Sitting. Sci Rep. 2017;7(1):6055.
- Warburton DER, et al. Health benefits of physical activity: the evidence. CMAJ. 2006 Mar;174(6):801-9.

CHAPTER 14 – CRY FOWL

- Aditi, Shariff M. Nipah virus infection: A review. Vol. 147, Epidemiology and Infection. Cambridge University Press; 2019.
- Astill J, et al. Detecting and predicting emerging disease in poultry with the implementation of new technologies and big data: A focus on avian influenza virus. Vol. 5, Frontiers in Veterinary Science. Frontiers Media S.A.; 2018. p. 263.
- Bennett CE, et al. The broiler chicken as a signal of a human reconfigured biosphere. R Soc Open Sci. 2018 Dec;5(12).
- Bintsis T. Foodborne pathogens. AIMS Microbiol. 2017;3(3):529-63.
- Campbell TC. Cancer prevention and treatment by wholistic nutrition. Journal of nature and science. 2017 Oct;3(10).
- Daniel CR, et al. Trends in meat consumption in the USA. Public Health Nutr. 2011 Apr;14(4):575-83.
- Davies R, Wales A. Antimicrobial Resistance on Farms: A Review Including Biosecurity and the Potential Role of Disinfectants in Resistance Selection. Vol. 18, Comprehensive Reviews in Food Science and Food Safety. Blackwell Publishing Inc.; 2019. p. 753-74.
- Dewey-Mattia D, et al. Surveillance for Foodborne Disease Outbreaks - United States, 2009-2015. MMWR Surveill Summ. 2018;67(10).
- Edwards CE, et al. Swine acute diarrhea syndrome coronavirus replication in primary human cells reveals potential susceptibility to infection. Proc Natl Acad Sci U S A. 2020 Oct;117(43):26915-25.
- Ganmaa D, Sato A. The possible role of female sex hormones in milk from pregnant cows in the development of breast, ovarian and corpus uteri cancers. Med Hypotheses. 2005;65(6):1028-37.
- https://www.economist.com/international/2019/01/19/how-chicken-became-the-rich-worlds-most-popular-meat
- https://www.sentienceinstitute.org/us-factory-farming-estimates
- Ito T. Wild birds and avian influenza. Journal of the Japanese Society on Poultry Diseases (Japan). 2007.
- Iwami S, et al. Avian flu pandemic: Can we prevent it? J Theor Biol. 2009 Mar;257(1):181-90.

- Jung K, et al. Porcine epidemic diarrhea virus (PEDV): An update on etiology, transmission, pathogenesis, and prevention and control. Vol. 286, Virus Research. Elsevier B.V.; 2020. p. 198045.
- Kahn CM, Line S, editors. The Merck veterinary manual. Kenilworth, NJ: Merck; 2010 Feb.
- Lekagul A, et al. Patterns of antibiotic use in global pig production: A systematic review. Vol. 7, Veterinary and Animal Science. Elsevier B.V.; 2019. p. 100058.
- Luo Y, et al. Broad Cell Tropism of SADS-CoV In Vitro Implies Its Potential Cross-Species Infection Risk. Virologica Sinica. Science Press; 2020. p. 1-5.
- Malekinejad H, Rezabakhsh A. Hormones in dairy foods and their impact on public health- A narrative review article. Iran J Public Health. 2015 Jun;44(6):742-58.
- Manyi-Loh C, et al. Antibiotic use in agriculture and its consequential resistance in environmental sources: Potential public health implications. Vol. 23, Molecules. MDPI AG; 2018.
- National Chicken Council. Per Capita Consumption of Poultry and Livestock, 1965 to Estimated 2021, in Pounds.
- Paxton H, et al. The gait dynamics of the modern broiler chicken: A cautionary tale of selective breeding. J Exp Biol. 2013 Sep;216(17):3237-48.
- Prestinaci F, et al. Antimicrobial resistance: A global multifaceted phenomenon. Vol. 109, Pathogens and Global Health. Maney Publishing; 2015. p. 309-18.
- Rossi J, Garner SA. Industrial Farm Animal Production: A Comprehensive Moral Critique. Vol. 27, Journal of Agricultural and Environmental Ethics. Kluwer Academic Publishers; 2014. p. 479-522.
- Rusu L, et al. Pesticide residues contamination of milk and dairy products. A case study: Bacau district area, Romania. J. Environ. Prot. Ecol. 2016 Jan 1;17:1229-41.
- Scallan E, et al. Foodborne illness acquired in the United States-Major pathogens. Emerg Infect Dis. 2011 Jan;17(1):7-15.
- Shi W, Gao GF. Emerging H5N8 avian influenza viruses. Science. 2021 May 21;372(6544):784-6.
- Viboud C, Simonsen L. Global mortality of 2009 pandemic influenza A H1N1. Vol. 12, The Lancet Infectious Diseases. Elsevier; 2012. p. 651-3.
- Wein Y, et al. Avoiding handling-induced stress in poultry: Use of uniform parameters to accurately determine physiological stress. Poult Sci. 2017 Jan;96(1):65-73.
- Yoon MY, Yoon SS. Disruption of the gut ecosystem by antibiotics. Vol. 59, Yonsei Medical Journal. Yonsei University College of Medicine; 2018. p. 4-12.
- Zuidhof MJ, et al. Growth, efficiency, and yield of commercial broilers from 1957, 1978, and 2005. Poult Sci. 2014 Dec;93(12):2970-82.

CHAPTER 15–PURGE YOUR PALATE

- Aguirre AA, et al. Illicit Wildlife Trade, Wet Markets, and COVID-19: Preventing Future Pandemics. World Med Heal Policy. 2020 Sep;12(3):256-65.
- Albrechtsen L, et al. Contrasts in availability and consumption of animal protein in Bioko Island, West Africa: The role of bushmeat. Environ Conserv. 2005;32(4):340-8.
- Aslam S, et al. Major risk factors for leprosy in a non-endemic area of the United States: A case series. IDCases. 2019 May;17:e00557-e00557.
- Bragagnolo C, et al. Hunting in Brazil: What are the options? Perspect Ecol Conserv. 2019;17(2):71-9.
- Campbell TC. Cancer prevention and treatment by wholistic nutrition. Journal of nature and science. 2017 Oct;3(10).
- Chan PKS. Outbreak of Avian Influenza A(H5N1) Virus Infection in Hong Kong in 1997. 2002. p. 58-64.
- Cox PA, Sacks OW. Cycad neurotoxins, consumption of flying foxes, and ALS-PDC disease in Guam. Neurology. 2002 Mar;58(6):956 LP - 959.
- D'Cruze N, et al. What is the true cost of the world's most expensive coffee? Oryx. 2014/03/13. 2014;48(2):170-1.
- da Silva MB, et al. Evidence of zoonotic leprosy in Pará, Brazilian Amazon, and risks associated with human contact or consumption of armadillos. PLoS Negl Trop Dis. 2018;12(6).
- El-Sayed A, Kamel M. Coronaviruses in humans and animals: the role of bats in viral evolution. Environ Sci Pollut Res. 2021;28(16):19589-600.
- Fa JE, et al. Bushmeat Exploitation in Tropical Forests: an Intercontinental Comparison. Conserv Biol. 2002 Feb;16(1):232-7.
- Goldberg TL, et al. Forest fragmentation as cause of bacterial transmission among nonhuman primates, humans, and livestock, Uganda. Emerg Infect Dis. 2008 Sep;14(9):1375-82.
- Han H-J, et al. Evidence for zoonotic origins of Middle East respiratory syndrome coronavirus. J Gen Virol. 2015/11/13. 2016 Feb;97(2):274-80.
- Hayman DTS, et al. Ebola virus antibodies in fruit bats, Ghana, West Africa. Emerg Infect Dis. 2012 Jul;18(7):1207-9.
- Jackson P. Fleshy Traffic, Feverish Borders: Blood, Birds, and Civet Cats in Cities Brimming with Intimate Commodities. 2008. p. 281-96.
- Jia G, et al. Fruit bats as a natural reservoir of zoonotic viruses. Chin Sci Bull. 2003;48(12):1179-82.
- Keenan SW, Elsey RM. The good, the bad, and the unknown: microbial symbioses of the American alligator. Integrative and comparative biology. 2015 Dec 1;55(6):972-85.
- Kerr-Pontes LRS, et al. Socioeconomic, environmental, and behavioural risk factors for leprosy in North-east Brazil: results of a case-control study. Int J Epidemiol. 2006 Aug;35(4):994-1000.
- Kurpiers LA, et al. Bushmeat and emerging infectious diseases: lessons from Africa. InProblematic wildlife 2016 (pp. 507-551). Springer, Cham.
- Leroy EM, et al. Fruit bats as reservoirs of Ebola virus. Nature. 2005;438(7068):575-6.
- Marcone MF. Composition and properties of Indonesian palm civet coffee (Kopi Luwak) and Ethiopian civet coffee. Food Res Int. 2004;37(9):901-12.
- Matos TS, et al. Leprosy in the elderly population and the occurrence of physical disabilities: Is there cause for concern? An Bras Dermatol. 2019/05/09. 2019;94(2):243-5.
- Moreno-Madriñán MJ, Turell M. History of Mosquitoborne Diseases in the United States and Implications for New Pathogens. Emerg Infect Dis. 2018 May;24(5):821-6.
- Naguib MM, et al. Live and Wet Markets: Food Access versus the Risk of Disease Emergence. Trends Microbiol. 2021 May;
- Nevarez JG, et al. Association of West Nile Virus with Lymphohistiocytic Proliferative Cutaneous Lesions in American Alligators. Zoo Wildl Med. 2008 Dec;39(4):562-6.
- Oliveira IVP de M, et al. Armadillos and leprosy: from infection to biological model. Rev Inst Med Trop Sao Paulo. 2019 Sep;61:e44-e44.
- Philippe Gaubert, et al. The Complete Phylogeny of Pangolins: Scaling Up Resources for the Molecular Tracing of the Most Trafficked Mammals on Earth. 2018. p. 247-359.
- Rewar S, Mirdha D. Transmission of Ebola Virus Disease: An Overview. Ann Glob Heal. 2014;80(6):444-51.
- Ripple WJ, et al. Bushmeat hunting and extinction risk to the world's mammals. R Soc Open Sci. 2016;3(10).
- Sharp PM, Hahn BH. Origins of HIV and the AIDS pandemic. Cold Spring Harb Perspect Med. 2011 Sep;1(1):a006841-a006841.
- Sunny B, et al. Maggot Infestation: Various Treatment Modalities. J Am Coll Clin Wound Spec. 2018 Mar;8(1-3):51-3.
- Wang LF, Eaton BT. Bats, civets and the emergence of SARS. Curr Top Microbiol Immunol. 2007;315:325-44.
- Wang Y, et al. Knowledge and attitudes about the use of pangolin scale products in Traditional Chinese Medicine (TCM) within China. People Nat . 2020 Dec;2(4):903-12.
- Wilkie DS, et al. Role of prices and wealth in consumer demand for bushmeat in Gabon, Central Africa. Conserv Biol. 2005;19(1):268-74.
- Zhang T, et al. Probable pangolin origin of SARS-CoV-2 associated with the COVID-19 outbreak. Current biology. 2020 Apr 6;30(7):1346-51.

CHAPTER 16 – INFECTION PROTECTION

- Aranow C. Vitamin D and the immune system. Journal of investigative medicine. 2011 Aug 1;59(6):881-6.
- Bennett JM, et al. Inflammation-nature's way to efficiently respond to all types of challenges: implications for understanding and managing "the epidemic" of chronic diseases. Frontiers in Medicine. 2018 Nov 27;5:316.
- Biesalski HK. Vitamin D deficiency and co-morbidities in COVID-19 patients-A fatal relationship?. Nfs Journal. 2020 Aug;20:10.
- Brower V. When the immune system goes on the attack: Thanks to advances in research, it may soon be easier to diagnose autoimmune diseases earlier, but therapy remains a tricky problem. EMBO reports. 2004 Aug;5(8):757-60.
- Clayton E, Munir M. Fundamental Characteristics of Bat Interferon Systems. Frontiers in cellular and infection microbiology. 2020 Dec 11;10:762.
- Cuzzocrea S, et al. Protective effects of N-acetylcysteine on lung injury and red blood cell modification induced by carrageenan in the rat. The FASEB Journal. 2001 May;15(7):1187-200.
- Fajgenbaum DC, June CH. Cytokine storm. New England Journal of Medicine. 2020 Dec 3;383(23):2255-73.
- Gammoh NZ, Rink L. Zinc in infection and inflammation. Nutrients. 2017 Jun;9(6):624.
- García-Sastre A. Ten strategies of interferon evasion by viruses. Cell host & microbe. 2017 Aug 9;22(2):176-84.
- Juybari KB, et al. Melatonin potentials against viral infections including COVID-19: Current evidence and new findings. Virus research. 2020 Aug 5:198108.
- Kimber I, Dearman RJ. Immune responses: adverse versus non-adverse effects. Toxicologic pathology. 2002 Jan;30(1):54-8.
- Le Page C, et al. Interferon activation and innate immunity. Reviews in immunogenetics. 2000 Jan 1;2(3):374-86.
- Lindsay B. The immune system. Nicholson Essays in Biochemistry. 2016 Oct 31;60:275-301.
- Liu Q, et al. Selenium (Se) plays a key role in the biological effects of some viruses: Implications for COVID-19. Environmental research. 2021 May 1;196:110984.
- Mahmudpour M, et al. COVID-19 cytokine storm: The anger of inflammation. Cytokine. 2020 May 30:155151.
- Mescher AL, Neff AW. Regenerative capacity and the developing immune system. Regenerative medicine I. 2005 Dec:39-66.
- Mokhtari V, et al. A review on various uses of N-acetyl cysteine. Cell Journal (Yakhteh). 2017 Apr;19(1):11.
- National Research Council (US) Committee on Research Opportunities in Biology. Opportunities in Biology. Washington (DC): National Academies Press (US); 1989. 7, The Immune System and Infectious Diseases.
- Ng WH, et al. Comorbidities in SARS-CoV-2 patients: a systematic review and meta-analysis. Mbio. 2021 Jan;12(1).
- Nguyen SV, et al. HIV blocks Type I IFN signaling through disruption of STAT1 phosphorylation. Innate immunity. 2018 Nov;24(8):490-500.
- Prather AA, et al. Temporal links between self-reported sleep and antibody responses to the influenza vaccine. International journal of behavioral medicine. 2021 Feb;28(1):151-8.
- Ramsey JM, et al. Atlas of Mexican Triatominae (Reduviidae: Hemiptera) and vector transmission of Chagas disease. Memórias do Instituto Oswaldo Cruz. 2015 May;110(3):339-52.
- Ryabkova VA, et al. Influenza infection, SARS, MERS and COVID-19: Cytokine storm-The common denominator and the lessons to be learned. Clinical Immunology. 2020 Dec 14:108652.
- Shi Z, Puyo CA. N-Acetylcysteine to Combat COVID-19: An Evidence Review. Therapeutics and clinical risk management. 2020;16:1047.
- Spiering MJ. Primer on the immune system. Alcohol research: current reviews. 2015;37(2):171.
- Taefehshokr N, et al. Covid-19: Perspectives on Innate Immune Evasion. Frontiers in immunology. 2020;11.
- Thomson CD, et al. Brazil nuts: an effective way to improve selenium status. The American journal of clinical nutrition. 2008 Feb 1;87(2):379-84.
- Traugott U, Lebon P. Multiple sclerosis: involvement of interferons in lesion pathogenesis. Annals of Neurology: Official Journal of the American Neurological Association and the Child Neurology Society. 1988 Aug;24(2):243-51.
- Zhang YY, et al. The comparative immunological characteristics of SARS-CoV, MERS-CoV, and SARS-CoV-2 coronavirus infections. Frontiers in Immunology. 2020 Aug 14;11:2033.
- Zhao J, et al. Evasion by stealth: inefficient immune activation underlies poor T cell response and severe disease in SARS-CoV-infected mice. PLoS Pathog. 2009 Oct 23;5(10):e1000636.

CHAPTER 17–GET OUT OF YOUR HEAD

- Bailey RR. Goal setting and action planning for health behavior change. American journal of lifestyle medicine. 2019 Nov;13(6):615-8.
- Bernecker K, Job V. Beliefs about willpower moderate the effect of previous day demands on next day's expectations and effective goal striving. Frontiers in Psychology. 2015 Oct 14;6:1496.
- Collazos CA, et al. Evaluating collaborative learning processes using system-based measurement. Educational Technology & Society. 2007 Apr;10(3):257-74.
- De Ridder D, Gillebaart M. Lessons learned from trait self-control in well-being: Making the case for routines and initiation as important components of trait self-control. Health psychology review. 2017 Jan 2;11(1):89-99.
- Feeney BC, Collins NL. Thriving through relationships. Current Opinion in Psychology. 2015 Feb 1;1:22-8.
- Gailliot MT, Baumeister RF. The physiology of willpower: Linking blood glucose to self-control. Personality and social psychology review. 2007 Nov;11(4):303-27.
- Gillebaart M. The 'operational'definition of self-control. Frontiers in psychology. 2018 Jul 18;9:1231.
- Lopez RB, et al. Neural mechanisms of emotion regulation and their role in endocrine and immune functioning: a review with implications for treatment of affective disorders. Neuroscience & Biobehavioral Reviews. 2018 Dec 1;95:508-14.
- Nedley N, Ramirez FE. Emotional Health and Stress Management. In Lifestyle Medicine 2019 Apr 17 (pp. 1003-1017). CRC Press.
- Oscar-Berman M, Marinković K. Alcohol: effects on neurobehavioral functions and the brain. Neuropsychology review. 2007 Sep 1;17(3):239-57.
- Rosen PJ, et al. Social self-control, externalizing behavior, and peer liking among children with ADHD-CT: A mediation model. Social Development. 2014 May;23(2):288-305.
- Snyder MA. Biblical Foundations for Nutrition and an Abundant Life. The Journal of Biblical Foundations of Faith and Learning. 2016;1(1):12.
- Sygit-Kowalkowska E, et al. Samokontrola emocjonalna, radzenie sobie ze stresem a samopoczucie psychofizyczne funkcjonariuszy służby więziennej [Emotional self-control, coping with stress and psycho-physical well-being of prison officers]. Med Pr. 2015;66(3):373-82.

CHAPTER 18–BRUSH YOUR TEETH

- Aas JA, et al. Defining the normal bacterial flora of the oral cavity. Journal of clinical microbiology. 2005 Nov;43(11):5721.
- Bergström J. Tobacco smoking and chronic destructive periodontal disease. Odontology. 2004 Sep;92(1):1-8.
- Blasi C. Iodine mouthwashes as deterrents against severe acute respiratory syndrome coronavirus 2 (SARS-CoV-2). Infection Control and Hospital Epidemiology. 2020.
- Deasy MJ, Vogel RI. Female sex hormonal factors in periodontal disease. Annals of dentistry. 1976;35(3):42-6.
- Eagappan AS, et al. Evaluation of salivary nitric oxide level in children with early childhood caries. Dental research journal. 2016 Jul;13(4):338.
- Eke PI, et al. Periodontitis in US Adults: National Health and Nutrition Examination Survey 2009-2014. Vol. 149, Journal of the American Dental Association. 2018. p. 576-588.e6.
- Gagari E, Kabani S. Adverse effects of mouthwash use. A review. Oral surgery, oral medicine, oral pathology, oral radiology, and endodontics. 1995 Oct 1;80(4):432-9.
- Ghapanchi J, et al. In vitro comparison of cytotoxic and antibacterial effects of 16 commercial toothpastes. [Internet]. Vol. 7, Journal of international oral health : JIOH. 2015. p. 39-43.
- Gürgan CA, et al. Short-term side effects of 0.2% alcohol-free chlorhexidine mouthrinse used as an adjunct to non-surgical periodontal treatment: a double-blind clinical study. J Periodontol. 2006;77(3):370-384.
- Hasani Tabatabaei M, et al. Cytotoxicity of the Ingredients of Commonly Used Toothpastes and Mouthwashes on Human Gingival Fibroblasts. Frontiers in Dentistry. 2020.
- Hoo GWS, et al. Fatal large-volume mouthwash ingestion in an adult: A review and the possible role of phenolic compound toxicity. Vol. 18, Journal of Intensive Care Medicine. 2003. p. 150-5.
- Kim J, Amar S. Periodontal disease and systemic conditions: a bidirectional relationship. Odontology. 2006 Sep;94(1):10-21.
- Lai AC, et al. Effectiveness of facemasks to reduce exposure hazards for airborne infections among general populations. Journal of the Royal Society Interface. 2012 May 7;9(70):938-48.
- Lv N, et al. Management of oral medicine emergencies during COVID-19: A study to develop practise guidelines. Journal of Dental Sciences. 2020.
- Marouf N, et al. Association between periodontitis and severity of COVID-19 infection: A case-control study. Journal of clinical periodontology. 2021 Apr 1;48(4):483-91.
- Michaud DS, et al. Periodontal disease, tooth loss, and cancer risk. Vol. 39, Epidemiologic Reviews. 2017. p. 49-58.
- Nazir MA. Prevalence of periodontal disease, its association with systemic diseases and prevention. Int J Health Sci (Qassim). 2017;11(2):72-80.
- Olsen I, Yamazaki K. Can oral bacteria affect the microbiome of the gut?. Journal of oral microbiology. 2019 Jan 1;11(1):1586422.
- Pinzan-Vercelino C, et al. Does the use of face masks during the COVID-19 pandemic impact on oral hygiene habits, oral conditions, reasons to seek dental care and esthetic concerns? Journal of Clinical and Experimental Dentistry. 2021. p. e369-75.
- Roberge RJ, et al. Physiological impact of the N95 filtering facepiece respirator on healthcare workers. Respiratory care. 2010 May 1;55(5):569-77.
- Sachdev R, et al. Is safeguard compromised? Surgical mouth mask harboring hazardous microorganisms in dental practice. Journal of family medicine and primary care. 2020 Feb;9(2):759.
- Sachdev R, et al. Is safeguard compromised? Surgical mouth mask harboring hazardous microorganisms in dental practice. Vol. 9, Journal of Family Medicine and Primary Care. 2020. p. 759.
- Scannapieco FA, Gershovich E. The prevention of periodontal disease–An overview. Periodontology 2000. 2020 Oct;84(1):9-13.
- Schiff T, et al. A clinical investigation of the efficacy of three different treatment regimens for the control of plaque and gingivitis. Vol. 17, Journal of Clinical Dentistry. 2006. p. 138-44.
- Schure NSGRS. Periodontal Disease - StatPearls - NCBI Bookshelf [Internet]. Ncbi. Available from: https://www.ncbi.nlm.nih.gov/books/NBK554590/
- Shang Q, et al. Interaction of oral and toothbrush microbiota affects oral cavity health. Frontiers in cellular and infection microbiology. 2020;10.
- Singh RK, et al. Influence of diet on the gut microbiome and implications for human health. Vol. 15, Journal of Translational Medicine. 2017.
- Smith JD, et al. Effectiveness of N95 respirators versus surgical masks in protecting health care workers from acute respiratory infection: a systematic review and meta-analysis. Cmaj. 2016 May 17;188(8):567-74.
- Tan C, et al. C-reactive protein correlates with computed tomographic findings and predicts severe COVID-19 early. Journal of medical virology. 2020 Jul;92(7):856-62.
- Tartaglia GM, et al. Adverse events associated with home use of mouthrinses: a systematic review. Vol. 10, Therapeutic Advances in Drug Safety. 2019.
- Tenelanda-López D, et al. Eating Habits and Their Relationship to Oral Health. Nutrients. 2020 Sep;12(9):2619.
- Vranic E, et al. Formulation ingredients for toothpastes and mouthwashes. Bosnian journal of basic medical sciences. 2004 Nov;4(4):51.
- Walia M, Saini N. Relationship between periodontal diseases and preterm birth: Recent epidemiological and biological data. International Journal of Applied and Basic Medical Research. 2015 Jan;5(1):2.
- Wang G, et al. C-Reactive Protein Level May Predict the Risk of COVID-19 Aggravation. Open Forum Infect Dis. 2020;7(5):ofaa153. Published 2020 Apr 29.
- Werner CD, Seymour RA. Are alcohol containing mouthwashes safe?. British dental journal. 2009 Nov;207(10):E19-.

CHAPTER 19–RECOVER YOUR JOY

- Beamish AJ, et al. What's in a smile? A review of the benefits of the clinician's smile. Vol. 95, Postgraduate Medical Journal. 2019. p. 91-5.
- Beetz A, et al. Psychosocial and psychophysiological effects of human-animal interactions: The possible role of oxytocin. Vol. 3, Frontiers in Psychology. 2012.
- Bennett MP, Lengacher C. Humor and Laughter May Influence Health [Part] IV. Humor and Immune Function.
- Buchowski MS, et al. Energy expenditure of genuine laughter. International journal of obesity. 2007 Jan;31(1):131-7.
- Byosiere SE, et al. Investigating the function of play bows in dog and Wolf Puppies (Canis lupus familiaris, Canis lupus occidentalis). Vol. 11, PLoS ONE. 2016.
- Collard RR. Fear of strangers and play behavior in kittens with varied social experience. Vol. 38, Child development. 1967. p. 877-91.
- Dochtermann NA, Jenkins SH. Behavioural syndromes in Merriam's kangaroo rats (Dipodomys merriami): A test of competing hypotheses. Vol. 274, Proceedings of the Royal Society B: Biological Sciences. 2007. p. 2343-9.
- Fagen RM. Salmonid jumping and playing: Potential cultural and welfare implications. Vol. 7, Animals. 2017.
- Fraser ON, Bugnyar T. The quality of social relationships in ravens. Vol. 79, Animal Behaviour. 2010. p. 927-33.
- Goumas M, et al. Herring gulls respond to human gaze direction. Vol. 15, Biology Letters. 2019.
- Ikeda H, et al. Social object play between captive bottlenose and Risso's dolphins. Vol. 13, PLoS ONE. 2018.
- Kaufmann JH. Field observations of the social behaviour of the eastern grey kangaroo, Macropus giganteus. Animal Behaviour. 1975 Feb 1;23:214-21.
- Ladds Z, et al. Social learning in otters. Vol. 4, Royal Society Open Science. 2017.
- Lee PC, Moss CJ. African elephant play, competence and social complexity. Animal Behavior and Cognition. 2014;1(2):144-56.
- Miller M, Fry WF. The effect of mirthful laughter on the human cardiovascular system. Medical hypotheses. 2009 Nov 1;73(5):636-9.

REFERENCES

- Moesta A, Crowell-Davis S. Intercat aggression - General considerations, prevention and treatment. Vol. 39, Tierarztliche Praxis Ausgabe K: Kleintiere - Heimtiere. 2011. p. 97-104.
- Morpurgo B, et al. Aggressive behaviour in immature captive Nile crocodiles, Crocodylus niloticus, in relation to feeding. Vol. 53, Physiology and Behavior. 1993. p. 1157-61.
- O Ogundele M. Behavioural and emotional disorders in childhood: A brief overview for paediatricians [Internet]. Vol. 7, World Journal of Clinical Pediatrics. 2018. p. 9-26. Available from: https://www.ncbi.nlm.nih.gov/pmc/articles/PMC5803568/pdf/WJCP-7-9.pdf
- Pinchover S. The relation between teachers' and children's playfulness: A pilot study. Vol. 8, Frontiers in Psychology. 2017.
- Proyer RT, et al. The positive relationships of playfulness with indicators of health, activity, and physical fitness. Vol. 9, Frontiers in Psychology. 2018.
- Schönfeld P, et al. The effects of daily stress on positive and negative mental health: Mediation through self-efficacy. Vol. 16, International Journal of Clinical and Health Psychology. 2016. p. 1-10.
- Seeman TE. Social ties and health: The benefits of social integration. Annals of epidemiology. 1996 Sep 1;6(5):442-51.
- Serafini G, et al. The psychological impact of COVID-19 on the mental health in the general population. QJM: An International Journal of Medicine. 2020 Aug 1;113(8):531-7.
- Siviy SM. A brain motivated to play: Insights into the neurobiology of playfulness. Vol. 153, Behaviour. 2016. p. 819-44.
- Snyder RJ, et al. Behavioral and Developmental Consequences of Early Rearing Experience for Captive Giant Pandas (Ailuropoda melanoleuca). Vol. 117, Journal of Comparative Psychology. 2003. p. 235-45.
- Tse MM, et al. Humor therapy: relieving chronic pain and enhancing happiness for older adults. Journal of aging research. 2010 Jun 28;2010.
- Umberson D, Karas Montez J. Social Relationships and Health: A Flashpoint for Health Policy. Vol. 51, Journal of Health and Social Behavior. 2010. p. S54-66.
- Yaribeygi H, et al. The impact of stress on body function: A review. Vol. 16, EXCLI Journal. 2017. p. 1057-72.

CHAPTER 20 — BATTLE THE BULGE

- Alperet DJ, et al. Influence of temperate, subtropical, and tropical fruit consumption on risk of type 2 diabetes in an Asian population. The American journal of clinical nutrition. 2017 Mar 1;105(3):736-45.
- Andersen CJ, et al. Impact of obesity and metabolic syndrome on immunity. Advances in Nutrition. 2016 Jan;7(1):66-75.
- Andersen DK. Diabetes and cancer: placing the association in perspective. Current Opinion in Endocrinology, Diabetes and Obesity. 2013 Apr 1;20(2):81-6.
- Carmody RN, et al. Cooking shapes the structure and function of the gut microbiome. Nature microbiology. 2019 Dec;4(12):2052-63.
- Catterson JH, et al. Short-term, intermittent fasting induces long-lasting gut health and TOR-independent lifespan extension. Current Biology. 2018 Jun 4;28(11):1714-24.
- Cercato C, Fonseca FA. Cardiovascular risk and obesity. Diabetology & metabolic syndrome. 2019 Dec;11(1):1-5.
- Chaput JP, Tremblay A. Adequate sleep to improve the treatment of obesity. Cmaj. 2012 Dec 11;184(18):1975-6.
- Chianese R, et al. Impact of dietary fats on brain functions. Current neuropharmacology. 2018 Aug 1;16(7):1059-85.
- Chiu CJ, et al. Association between dietary glycemic index and age-related macular degeneration in nondiabetic participants in the Age-Related Eye Disease Study. The American journal of clinical nutrition. 2007 Jul 1;86(1):180-8.
- Choi YJ, et al. An exploratory study on the effect of daily fruits and vegetable juice on human gut microbiota. Food science and biotechnology. 2018 Oct;27(5):1377-86.
- Chon TJ, et al. Enhancing psychological and physical fitness factors of Korea middle school students by introducing rope skipping. Vol. 47, Iranian Journal of Public Health. 2018. p. 1965-6.
- Clar C, et al. Low glycaemic index diets for the prevention of cardiovascular disease. Cochrane Database of Systematic Reviews. 2017(7).
- de Siqueira JV, et al. Impact of obesity on hospitalizations and mortality, due to COVID-19: a systematic review. Obesity research & clinical practice. 2020 Jul 23.
- Ding C, et al. Lean, but not healthy: the 'metabolically obese, normal-weight'phenotype. Current opinion in clinical nutrition and metabolic care. 2016 Nov 1;19(6):408-17.
- Eldin IM, et al. Preliminary study of the clinical hypoglycemic effects of Allium cepa (red onion) in type 1 and type 2 diabetic patients. Environmental health insights. 2010 Jan;4:EHI-S5540.
- Eleazu CO. The concept of low glycemic index and glycemic load foods as panacea for type 2 diabetes mellitus; prospects, challenges and solutions. African health sciences. 2016 Jul 1;16(2):468-79.
- Evans DR, et al. The Nature of Self-Regulatory Fatigue and "Ego Depletion": Lessons From Physical Fatigue. Vol. 20, Personality and Social Psychology Review. 2016. p. 291-310.
- Golay A, Ybarra J. Link between obesity and type 2 diabetes. Best Pract Res Clin Endocrinol Metab. 2005 Dec;19(4):649-63.
- Heymsfield SB, et al. Why are there race/ethnic differences in adult body mass index–adiposity relationships? A quantitative critical review. Obesity reviews. 2016 Mar;17(3):262-75.
- Hruby A, Hu FB. The Epidemiology of Obesity: A Big Picture. Vol. 33, Pharmacoeconomics. 2015. p. 673-89.
- Iannelli A, et al. Obesity and COVID-19: ACE 2, the missing tile. Obesity Surgery. 2020 Nov;30:4615-7.
- Iglesias Molli AE, et al. Metabolically healthy obese individuals present similar chronic inflammation level but less insulin-resistance than obese individuals with metabolic syndrome. PLoS One. 2017 Dec 28;12(12):e0190528.
- Ilich JZ, et al. Osteosarcopenic obesity syndrome: what is it and how can it be identified and diagnosed?. Current gerontology and geriatrics research. 2016 Oct;2016.
- Jenkins DJ, et al. Effect of legumes as part of a low glycemic index diet on glycemic control and cardiovascular risk factors in type 2 diabetes mellitus: a randomized controlled trial. Archives of internal medicine. 2012 Nov 26;172(21):1653-60.
- Keithley JK, Swanson B. Glucomannan and obesity: a critical review. Alternative therapies in health and medicine. 2005 Nov 1;11(6):30-5.
- Kim DY, et al. Effect of walking exercise on changes in cardiorespiratory fitness, metabolic syndrome markers, and high-molecular-weight adiponectin in obese middle-aged women. Journal of physical therapy science. 2014;26(11):1723-7.
- Kompaniyets L, et al. Body mass index and risk for COVID-19-related hospitalization, intensive care unit admission, invasive mechanical ventilation, and death–united states, march–december 2020. Morbidity and Mortality Weekly Report. 2021 Mar 12;70(10):355.
- Liu AG, et al. A healthy approach to dietary fats: understanding the science and taking action to reduce consumer confusion. Nutrition journal. 2017 Dec;16(1):1-5.
- Lo HC, Wasser SP. Medicinal mushrooms for glycemic control in diabetes mellitus: history, current status, future perspectives, and unsolved problems. International journal of medicinal mushrooms. 2011;13(5).
- Magliano M. Obesity and arthritis. Menopause International. 2008 Dec;14(4):149-54.
- McKay NJ, et al. Increasing water intake influences hunger and food preference, but does not reliably suppress energy intake in adults. Physiology & behavior. 2018 Oct 1;194:15-22.
- Milner JJ, Beck MA. The impact of obesity on the immune response to infection. Proceedings of the Nutrition Society. 2012 May;71(2):298-306.
- Mohammadi-Sartang M, et al. The effect of flaxseed supplementation on body weight and body composition: a systematic review and meta-analysis of 45 randomized placebo-controlled trials. Obesity Reviews. 2017 Sep;18(9):1096-107.
- Moller L, et al. Impact of fasting on growth hormone signaling and action in muscle and fat. The Journal of Clinical Endocrinology & Metabolism. 2009 Mar 1;94(3):965-72.
- Ng M, et al. Global, regional, and national prevalence of overweight and obesity in children and adults during 1980–2013: a systematic analysis for the Global Burden of Disease Study 2013,,. The Lancet. 2014;384(9945):766-81.
- Ntzouvani A, et al. Effects of nut and seed consumption on markers of glucose metabolism in adults with prediabetes: a systematic review of randomised controlled trials. British Journal of Nutrition. 2019 Aug;122(4):361-75.
- Ofei F. Obesity-a preventable disease. Ghana medical journal. 2005 Sep;39(3):98.
- Paoli A, et al. The influence of meal frequency and timing on health in humans: the role of fasting. Nutrients. 2019 Apr;11(4):719.
- Pasquali R, et al. Obesity and infertility. Current Opinion in Endocrinology, Diabetes, and Obesity. 2007 Dec 1;14(6):482-7.
- Philippou E, Constantinou M. The influence of glycemic index on cognitive functioning: a systematic review of the evidence. Advances in Nutrition. 2014 Mar;5(2):119-30.
- Popkin BM, et al. Water, hydration, and health. Nutr Rev. 2010 Aug;68(8):439-58.
- Radulian G, et al. Metabolic effects of low glycaemic index diets. Nutrition journal. 2009 Dec;8(1):1-8.
- Rodríguez-Hernández H, et al. Obesity and inflammation: epidemiology, risk factors, and markers of inflammation. International journal of endocrinology. 2013 Oct;2013.
- Slavin JL, Lloyd B. Health benefits of fruits and vegetables. Adv Nutr 2012; 3 (4): 506-516.
- Smith LW, et al. Involvement of nitric oxide synthase in skeletal muscle adaptation to chronic overload. Journal of Applied Physiology. 2002 May 1;92(5):2005-11.
- Templeman I, et al. Intermittent fasting, energy balance and associated health outcomes in adults: study protocol for a randomised controlled trial. Trials. 2018 Dec;19(1):1-1.
- Thornton SN. Increased hydration can be associated with weight loss. Frontiers in nutrition. 2016 Jun 10;3:18.
- Truswell AS. Glycaemic index of foods. European Journal of Clinical Nutrition. 1992 Oct 1;46:S91-101.
- Turati F, et al. Glycemic index, glycemic load and cancer risk: an updated meta-analysis. Nutrients. 2019 Oct;11(10):2342.
- Vogel P, et al. Polyphenols benefits of olive leaf (Olea europaea L) to human health. Nutrición hospitalaria. 2015;31(3):1427-33.
- Wang PY, et al. Higher intake of fruits, vegetables or their fiber reduces the risk of type 2 diabetes: a meta-analysis. J Diabetes Investig 2016; 7: 56-69.
- Weir CB, Jan A. BMI classification percentile and cut off points. StatPearls [Internet]. 2019 Dec 7.
- Who EC. Appropriate body-mass index for Asian populations and its implications for policy and intervention strategies.[see comment][erratum appears in Lancet. 2004 Mar 13; 363 (9412): 902].[Review][31 refs]. Lancet. 2004;363(9403):157-63.
- Zafar MI, et al. Low-glycemic index diets as an intervention for diabetes: a systematic review and meta-analysis. The American journal of clinical nutrition. 2019 Oct 1;110(4):891-902.

- Zaragozano JF, et al. Psyllium fibre and the metabolic control of obese and adolescents. Journal of physiology and biochemistry. 2003;59(3):235-42.
- Zhao QM, et al. Global, regional and national prevalence of overweight and obesity in children and adults 1980-2013: A systematic analysis. Vol. 384, Europe PMC Funders Group Author Manuscript. 2020. p. 766-81.

CHAPTER 21 — REST FROM DISTRESS

- Aronson J, et al. Unhealthy interactions: The role of stereotype threat in health disparities. American journal of public health. 2013 Jan;103(1):50-6.
- Bail CA, et al. A. Exposure to opposing views on social media can increase political polarization. Proceedings of the National Academy of Sciences. 2018 Sep 11;115(37):9216-21.
- Balcetis E, Dunning D. See what you want to see: motivational influences on visual perception. Journal of personality and social psychology. 2006 Oct;91(4):612.
- Bjureberg J, Gross JJ. Regulating road rage. Social and personality psychology compass. 2021 Mar;15(3):e12586.
- Burns D. Feeling Good: The New Mood Therapy. New York, NY: Quill; 2000.
- Caouette JD, Guyer AE. Cognitive distortions mediate depression and affective response to social acceptance and rejection. Journal of affective disorders. 2016 Jan 15;190:792-9.
- Chand SP, et al. Cognitive Behavior Therapy. [Updated 2021 Apr 19]. In: StatPearls [Internet]. Treasure Island (FL): StatPearls Publishing; 2021 Jan-
- Cruz N, et al. Explaining away, augmentation, and the assumption of independence. Frontiers in Psychology. 2020;11:2721.
- Festinger L. Cognitive dissonance. Sci Am. 1962 Oct;207:93-102.
- Gilbert P. The evolved basis and adaptive functions of cognitive distortions. British Journal of Medical Psychology. 1998 Dec;71(4):447-63.
- Gregory Jr VL. Cognitive-Behavioral Therapy for Relationship Distress: Meta-analysis of RCTs with Social Work Implications. Journal of Evidence-Based Social Work. 2021 Jan 2;18(1):49-70.
- Harmer B, et al. Suicidal Ideation. 2021 Apr 28. In: StatPearls [Internet]. Treasure Island (FL): StatPearls Publishing; 2021 Jan-. PMID: 33351435.
- Haslam C, et al. Patients' experiences of medication for anxiety and depression: effects on working life. Family Practice. 2004 Apr 1;21(2):204-12.
- Jager-Hyman S, et al. Cognitive distortions and suicide attempts. Cognitive therapy and research. 2014 Aug 1;38(4):369-74.
- Jung N, et al. How emotions affect logical reasoning: evidence from experiments with mood-manipulated participants, spider phobics, and people with exam anxiety. Frontiers in psychology. 2014 Jun 10;5:570.
- Kelly JD. Your Best Life: Perfectionism—The Bane of Happiness. Clinical Orthopaedics and Related Research®. 2015 Oct;473(10):3108-11.
- Laufer O, et al. Behavioral and neural mechanisms of overgeneralization in anxiety. Current Biology. 2016 Mar 21;26(6):713-22.
- Lawler KA, et al. A change of heart: Cardiovascular correlates of forgiveness in response to interpersonal conflict. Journal of behavioral medicine. 2003 Oct;26(5):373-93.
- MacLeod AK, Williams JM. Overgeneralization: An important but non-homogeneous construct. British journal of clinical psychology. 1990 Nov;29(4):443-4.
- Moncrieff J, et al. The psychoactive effects of psychiatric medication: the elephant in the room. Journal of psychoactive drugs. 2013 Nov 1;45(5):409-15.
- Naylor E V., Antonuccio DO, Litt M, Johnson GE, Spogen DR, Williams R, et al. Bibliotherapy as a treatment for depression in primary care. Vol. 17, Journal of Clinical Psychology in Medical Settings. 2010. p. 258-71.
- Özdel K, et al. Measuring cognitive errors using the Cognitive Distortions Scale (CDS): Psychometric properties in clinical and non-clinical samples. PloS one. 2014 Aug 29;9(8):e105956.
- Ready CB, et al. Overgeneralized beliefs, accommodation, and treatment outcome in youth receiving trauma-focused cognitive behavioral therapy for childhood trauma. Behavior therapy. 2015 Sep 1;46(5):671-88.
- Robinson OJ, Vytal K, Cornwell BR, Grillon C. The impact of anxiety upon cognition: perspectives from human threat of shock studies. Vol. 7, Frontiers in Human Neuroscience. 2013.
- Rosner R, et al. Treatment of complicated grief. European journal of psychotraumatology. 2011 Jan 1;2(1):7995.
- Sanivarapu S. Black & white thinking: A cognitive distortion. Indian journal of psychiatry. 2015 Jan;57(1):94.
- Schulz P, Hede V. Alternative and complementary approaches in psychiatry: beliefs versus evidence. Dialogues in clinical neuroscience. 2018 Sep;20(3):207.
- Seligman ME. Authentic happiness: Using the new positive psychology to realize your potential for lasting fulfillment. Simon and Schuster; 2004.
- Seligman ME. Learned helplessness. Annual review of medicine. 1972 Feb;23(1):407-12.
- Staicu ML, Cuțov M. Anger and health risk behaviors. J Med Life. 2010 Oct-Dec;3(4):372-5.
- Stanisławski K. The coping circumplex model: an integrative model of the structure of coping with stress. Frontiers in psychology. 2019 Apr 16;10:694.
- Thomas G, Fletcher GJ. Mind-reading accuracy in intimate relationships: assessing the roles of the relationship, the target, and the judge. Journal of personality and social psychology. 2003 Dec;85(6):1079.
- Tilghman-Osborne C, Cole DA, Felton JW. Inappropriate and excessive guilt: Instrument validation and developmental differences in relation to depression. Vol. 40, Journal of Abnormal Child Psychology. 2012. p. 607-20.
- Velten J, et al. Lifestyle choices and mental health: a longitudinal survey with German and Chinese students. BMC Public Health. 2018 Dec;18(1):1-5.
- Vogeley K, et al. Mind reading: neural mechanisms of theory of mind and self-perspective. Neuroimage. 2001 Jul 1;14(1):170-81.

CHAPTER 22 — CHOOSE PEACE

- Andrade C, Radhakrishnan R. Prayer and healing: A medical and scientific perspective on randomized controlled trials. Indian journal of psychiatry. 2009 Jul;51(4):247.
- Belvederi Murri M, et al. Physical exercise in major depression: reducing the mortality gap while improving clinical outcomes. Frontiers in psychiatry. 2019 Jan 10;9:762.
- Brown J, et al. Spirituality and optimism: a holistic approach to component-based, self-management treatment for HIV. Journal of religion and health. 2014 Oct;53(5):1317-28.
- Brown RP, et al. Breathing practices for treatment of psychiatric and stress-related medical conditions. Psychiatric Clinics. 2013 Mar 1;36(1):121-40.
- Conversano C, et al. Optimism and its impact on mental and physical well-being. Clinical Practice & Epidemiology in Mental Health.;6(1):25-9.
- Hecht D. The neural basis of optimism and pessimism. Experimental neurobiology. 2013 Sep;22(3):173.
- Kim ES, et al. Optimism and cause-specific mortality: a prospective cohort study. American journal of epidemiology. 2017 Jan 1;185(1):21-9.
- Koeing HG. Religion, spirituality, and health: The research and clinical implications. International Scholarly Research Network. 2012;2012:278730.
- Lee LO, et al. Optimism is associated with exceptional longevity in 2 epidemiologic cohorts of men and women. Proceedings of the National Academy of Sciences. 2019 Sep 10;116(37):18357-62.
- Maratos A, et al. Music therapy for depression. Cochrane database of systematic reviews. 2008(1).
- Mårtensson B, et al. Bright white light therapy in depression: a critical review of the evidence. Journal of Affective Disorders. 2015 Aug 15;182:1-7.
- Mooventhan A, Nivethitha L. Scientific evidence-based effects of hydrotherapy on various systems of the body. North American journal of medical sciences. 2014 May;6(5):199.
- Nedley N, Ramirez FE. Nedley depression hit hypothesis: identifying depression and its causes. American journal of lifestyle medicine. 2016 Nov;10(6):422-8.
- Räikkönen K, et al. Effects of optimism, pessimism, and trait anxiety on ambulatory blood pressure and mood during everyday life. Journal of personality and social psychology. 1999 Jan;76(1):104.
- Scheier MF, Carver CS. Dispositional optimism and physical health: A long look back, a quick look forward. American Psychologist. 2018 Dec;73(9):1082.
- Segerstrom SC. Optimism and immunity: Do positive thoughts always lead to positive effects?. Brain, behavior, and immunity. 2005 May 1;19(3):195-200.
- Sharma S, et al. Reliability and path length analysis of irregular fault tolerant multistage interconnection network. ACM SIGARCH Computer Architecture News. 2010 Apr 6;37(5):16-23.
- Tausk F, et al. Psychoneuroimmunology. Dermatol Ther. 2008 Jan-Feb;21(1):22-31.
- Wesley J. The Journal of John Wesley. CH Kelly; 1903.
- Zhai L, et al. Sleep duration and depression among adults: A meta-analysis of prospective studies. Depression and anxiety. 2015 Sep;32(9):664-70.